D0094406

The
Magick
of
Aromatherapy

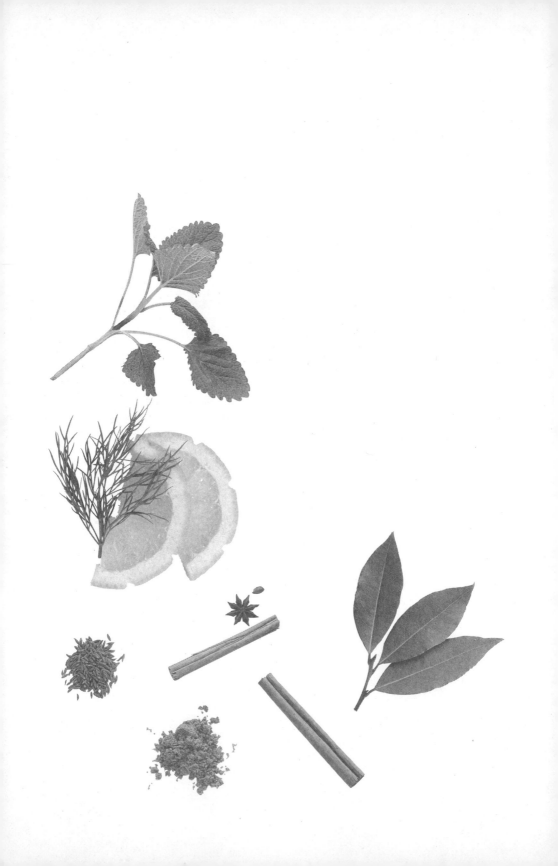

The Complete Guide for the Fragrance Artist

Learn to create blends of essential oils to better body, mind, and spirit! Based on the author's 20 years of research and experimentation, you'll get hundreds of time-tested recipes. Plus, discover for the first time how the art of aromatherapy has evolved into its present-day form.

The easy-to-follow recipes and the comprehensive reference section make *The Magick of Aromatherapy* perfect for both beginners and seasoned practitioners.

- Learn how to blend your own oils for the purposes of protection, love, and money
- Learn the therapeutic and magickal properties of a variety of scents
- Discover the two types of magickal workings
- Become familiar with the universal energies of elements and plants and how they influence aromatherapy
- Honor the gods and goddesses through scent
- Discover the mythological, historical, and contemporary uses of scents
- Learn the proper way to blend oils using major, minor, and trace influences

About the Author

Gwydion O'Hara has been a student of the natural arts and sciences for over twenty years. His research has been aimed at reclaiming the knowledge of our ancestors that has become obscured by time. This volume, the culmination of many years of research and study, is yet another exercise in recovering the beloved insights of our ancestors—those who sought and appreciated the gifts of nature.

To Write to the Author

If you wish to contact the author or would like more information about this book, please write to the author in care of Llewellyn Worldwide and we will forward your request. Both the author and publisher appreciate hearing from you and learning of your enjoyment of this book and how it has helped you. Llewellyn Worldwide cannot guarantee that every letter written to the author can be answered, but all will be forwarded. Please write to:

Gwydion O'Hara
℅ Llewellyn Worldwide
P.O. Box 64383, Dept. K348-4
St. Paul, MN 55164–0383, U.S.A.

Please enclose a self-addressed stamped envelope for reply,
or $1.00 to cover costs. If outside U.S.A., enclose international
postal reply coupon.

GWYDION O'HARA

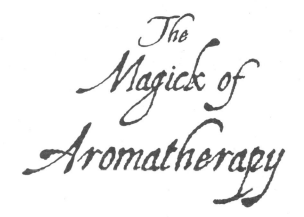

The
Magick of
Aromatherapy

The Use

of Scent for

Healing

Body,

Mind, and Spirit

1998
Llewellyn Publications
St. Paul, MN 55164-0383, U.S.A.

FIRST EDITION
First Printing, 1998

Cover design by Lisa Novak
Editing and book design by Rebecca Zins

Library of Congress Cataloging-in-Publication Data
O'Hara, Gwydion.
    The magick of aromatherapy: the use of scent for healing body, mind, and spirit / Gwydion O'Hara.—1st ed.
        p.   cm.
    Includes bibliographical references and index.
    Contents: Bare d'essence—Magick and healing with aromatherapy, book II.
    ISBN 1-56718-348-4 (trade paper)
    1. Aromatherapy.   I. O'Hara, Gwydion. Bare d'essence.
II. O'Hara, Gwydion. Magick and healing with aromatherapy, book II.
III. Title.
RM666.A68037   1998
615' .321—dc21   97-32117
                                                                                CIP

Llewellyn Worldwide does not participate in, endorse, or have any authority or responsibility concerning private business transactions between our authors and the public.
    All mail addressed to the author is forwarded but the publisher cannot, unless specifically instructed by the author, give out an address or phone number.

Llewellyn Publications
A Division of Llewellyn Worldwide, Ltd.
P.O. Box 64383, Dept. K348-4
St. Paul, MN 55164-0383, U.S.A.

Other Books by Gwydion O'Hara

Pagan Ways

Sun Lore

Moon Lore

For magicians, healers, herbalists,
aromatherapists, and lovers of the earth's
natural treasures. For those who seek to gain
the knowledge, the hidden sense of scents,
the essence of essentials.

Also dedicated to the memory of Herman Slater—

Vastly knowledgeable,
Deeply honored,
And delightfully opinionated.

We miss your voice, but cherish your memory.

Contents

PART III: SPIRIT
Essences of Aromatherapy

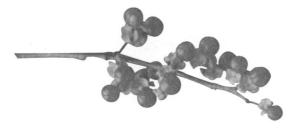

Acknowledgments

The Magick of Aromatherapy is the culmination of more than twenty years' research and experience in the field of herbology and essential oils. Along the way, in this or any other field of endeavor, no one works alone. There have been many who have given their knowledge, their insights, and their inspiration. In particular, Richard and Tamarra James of The Occult Shop in Toronto taught me much about oil blends, encouraged me to develop and follow my own instincts, and gave me the opportunity to experiment and play with a full complement of essential scents. Thanks also to Michele DiLeo for showing me how to bring a unique, living quality to any mixture.

Additionally, this book is a combination of traditional folklore formulas as well as new ideas spurred by needs as they have arisen. Thanks goes to many shop owners and individuals throughout Dallas-Ft. Worth for allowing me the opportunity to satisfy their customers' needs with newly created oil blends, for contributing many fresh ideas for the creation of scent, and for their continued friendship, support, and enthusiasm.

Preface

With the increasing interest in the natural arts and sciences, many have found a keen attraction to the workings of fragrance. There have been untold volumes published on the healing applications of scent, yet the magickal applications have been less celebrated. This is unfortunate, for two reasons. First, the magickal applications of aromatherapy—existing since before recorded history in the sacred rites of our ancestors, who burned herbs and essences to their deities—in many ways may have been the foundation of the rich healing practices of the modern-day aromatherapist. We can only expand our understanding of the art if we remember its roots. Secondly, and perhaps even more importantly, is the fact that the magickal practice of aromatherapy is inseparable from the therapeutic. The treatment of mind and spirit is a key concern of magickal endeavor. In treating many ailments, the healer has discovered that the mind and spirit of the client colors the effectiveness of a given remedy.

Although there may be those who look at the magickal applications of the fragrance arts as just so much superstition, as the old wives' tales of an ignorant world, it should be remembered that the folk remedies of our ancestors do indeed have substance. If we are truly a generation of wisdom and insight, we should not be too quick to dismiss the old magick. The lore that has been handed down from ancient days is but a piece of knowledge that was at one time necessary for "old wives" to know.

There is no shortage of available material on the art and science of aromatherapy. While some involved in working with fragrances fancy themselves artists—with a kinship to the perfumer of old, with a touch of elegance—others align themselves more closely with the medical practitioners and the scientific community. In order to fully explore the incredible world of scent, it is necessary to abandon classifications and to become open to the world of knowledge before us in whatever guise it may present itself.

The approach I have taken in dealing with this subject matter is one of open exploration and adventurous, uninhibited experimentation. By no means have I taken the mindset of the purist—and I invite you to follow my example. I take my lessons where I may, plunge deeply into the scented gifts of nature, and augment this world of wonder with the innovations created by the human mind.

Some will steer clear of anything "unnatural" in the practice of aromatherapy. Yet there appears to be an entire world of possibility abandoned with this approach. And if there is some level of justification required by the purist to ease the sense of betraying the natural order as I pursue the effects of synthetic aromas as well as those that occur in nature, consider the age-old use of a remedy like white willow bark as the predecessor to the common aspirin. What volume of white willow bark would be required to accomplish the same symptomatic relief as one tiny aspirin? And to further champion the use of natural as well as synthetic scents, cannot all substances find their beginnings in nature?

If the human mind can develop a way to enhance the effectiveness of nature's gifts, then I will not ignore the possibilities. For human thought is a creation of the natural order as well. To deny the pursuit of knowledge might be considered as much a betrayal of nature as our straying from the confines of aromas that are derived strictly from raw materials in their natural state. For in aromatherapy, we do not attempt to mutilate the gifts of nature, but rather to appreciate and utilize them to their fullest capacity.

Why Aromatherapy?

With all the available alternative healing methods available, what would make the art of the aromatherapist any more popular than another? Though there may be many different answers to this proposition, one that may be especially worthy of consideration is that of versatility. Within the scope of the oils that are the tools of the aromatherapy technician lies a world of possibility. Not only does each individual essential fragrance have virtues of its own, but the number of possible blends that may utilize the properties of several essentials is only limited by the knowledge and creative artistry of the person mixing them.

Blending fragrances to a specific healing purpose offers some facilities that are less apparent in other forms of alternative treatments. Taken from the expertise of the master perfumer is the use of the trace element in blends. While there may be only a drop or two of a particular essential oil included in a formula, this inclusion has the effect of totally altering the properties of the final blended product. It can increase the potency of a particular remedy or direct its effectiveness along specific lines of treatment, thus enhancing its overall potency.

Another virtue of using oil blends in healing pursuits is the employment of subtlety. While many of the healing arts approach the relief of symptoms or the attack of the causal bacteria of an ailment, aromatherapy has the ability to address treatment on more than one level. It can be directed toward relief of the symptoms of an ailment—used as a medium for cleansing and disinfecting, for ousting the offending microorganism. However, it may also be used as a catalyst to spur on the body's own natural defenses. It can be used to invoke and enhance the natural immune system, so that it kicks in at full power to alleviate the pain and suffering of an ailment. While it can parallel the successes of allo-pathic medicine, it may also be used as the homeopathy of alternative systems. It is the culmination of many centuries of research and experience, the best of many worlds.

One of the primary purposes of this volume is to open up the world of aroma to the individual, to expose each man and woman to a heightened awareness of the subtle conditions existing all around them that may have a significant effect upon their well-being. Whether the sensitivities are awakened by the fragrance of a field of wildflowers or of a manufactured perfumer's creation, whether one is assaulted by the odor of a stinkbug fallen beneath the shoe of a careless passerby or the penetrating stench of a chemical fire, you are affected by the scents you experience. In pursuing the spheres of fragrance, you will become more aware of your day-to-day experiences with scent, entering your future experiences with your eyes—and nostrils—wide open.

While there are many published works that may serve as formularies in aromatherapy, few address both the magickal and the healing aspects of the practice. And while this formulary may be one of the most expansive volumes presently available, it should be remembered that the possibilities of varying oil blends is endless, bound only by the expertise and creativity of the individual aromatherapist. Let this book serve as a guide to the gifts of nature—to use them to make your life better, your body healthier, and your mind and spirit robust with vitality.

Introduction

Long ago, when humankind struggled through a strange world in ignorance, there was no true science—perhaps, in those days of darkness, there was no true knowledge either. The races of people were as children upon the earth, struggling to make their way through each successive day to see the dawning of just one more sun. It was in this time that superstition gripped the minds of civilized beings, when popular belief stood in the place that was to be reserved for science and art as the wheel of time progressed.

Now we have fine health care facilities throughout the world to maintain our physical and mental well-being. There are medical remedies for almost every conceivable ailment and chemical concoctions devoted to every purpose. And yet the old-world beliefs have not completely faded from our lives. The superstitious world of civilization in its age of ignorance has taken a stubborn foothold in a new age of science and knowledge.

We know, now, that the world is not the center of the universe, as the pseudo-scientists of ages past would have had us believe. These one-time scholars of darkness—the astrologers, philosophers, and alchemists—have been proven wrong in many instances. Yet we pick up the daily newspaper and still consult the ancient systems of art and science as we peruse our daily horoscope. The old wives' tales are deeply rooted in cultures and family heritages; we swear by Granny's cold remedy that she inherited from her own Granny, and a hundred Grannys before her.

What is the obsession with the old beliefs that seems so inescapable in a modern world? While it may be true that science has overturned many of the old beliefs, it has given credibility to so many more. Mother's chicken soup has been found to contain a natural antibiotic that helps us to combat disease. The garlic that our ancestors were so fond of swallowing to chase away the demons that caused human suffering has also been found to have bacteria-fighting properties.

A dear friend once told me to not disregard the lore that has come down from distant years, for it often contained great wisdom. Within the substance of this simple statement is the foundation of the survival, and constant revival, of the ancient arts. Necessity was the motivation behind the old ways of healing. Centuries ago, as early as the year 1210, it was heralded that 'Nede makith the old wiff to trotte.' This proverb, as recorded in *The Common-place Book* before 1500, illuminates the driving force behind ancient home remedies and, perhaps, explains the reason for the successes of our ancestors in the healing arts. Their remedies had to be effective for their survival. They were not reaching for a Nobel prize; rather, the fruit of their labor was life itself.

And so the old arts continue to survive. Researchers are forever reaching back to ages past in hopes of touching one or another of the ancient magicks of our ancestors, whose many specks of light pierced the darkened world of ignorance before the dawn of science.

The use of scent for healing body, mind, and spirit was but one of those specks of illumination. Some of us may remember the smell of camphor that filled the room as Grandma took up the battle against winter colds on our behalf, or the smell of mustard used in the paste that heated our bodies and chased the congestion from our chests. There is a crossover between the herbal remedies of the country folk and the modern application of aromatherapy today. Just as the body may absorb medication through external application or direct ingestion, we take in the therapeutic value of our healing concoctions through their scent as it is absorbed by the sensitive membranes of our nasal passages.

The avid cocaine user and the abuser of inhalant substances know well the ability of the nasal membranes to absorb both scent and substance into the body. The aromatherapist employs the same principle for positive purpose, building and healing instead of weakening and tearing down.

Although the practice of aromatherapy has grown in popularity and usage over the past several decades, its effectiveness and its subtle workings have never required the attention of humankind. Whether we like it or not, or even choose to believe it or not, we are all subject to the effects created by our surroundings. We respond in different ways to color, to temperature, to the many sounds that fill our world—and we are no less affected by the smells we encounter each day.

When we inhale the fresh aroma of newly baked bread, the thought of tasting the hot loaves flows naturally through our minds. We need not even be hungry for the aroma to exercise its magick on us. The sweet scent of a field of flowers may fill us with peaceful, dreamy feelings—as well as evoke memories or fantasies from days gone by. As we journey through our everyday lives, we cannot be unaffected by the sensual stimuli of the scents we meet on our way.

The most obvious and sensually stirring scents are those that are unusual. Perhaps from our city dwelling we go to visit a rural area and are taken by the smell of the newly mown hay or assaulted by the gamey, piercing odor of the pig barn. In a strange setting, every smell seems to linger a bit longer in our nostrils. We breathe in deeply, fascinated by the aromas that surround us in this alien world. Every scent, the foul as well as the pleasant, holds a fascination for us, stimulating and exciting every fiber of our sensual perception.

Yet we are more often in the company of the familiar environment of our everyday existences. After experiencing the stimulating effect of the aromas that are new to us, it is inconceivable that we are not equally affected by the smells that permeate our own world. And, in fact, we are. Our constant exposure to the scents of our everyday lives, however, force their effect onto a subconscious level. If we were to stop and analyze each of the scents that we pass in our everyday existence, we might set out on a simple journey, perhaps to the corner store, and become hopelessly lost in a sea of sensual wonder. So we learn to place the stimuli of our everyday lives into subconscious acknowledgment so that we can get on with our daily tasks.

Consider, for example, the classic scene of the elderly soul who adores cats. It seems that almost everyone with whom I've ever spoken has had contact with such a figure in their own experience. Caring, compassionate, and appreciative of their company, the cat lover's animals are well tended and continue to multiply. It is difficult to have a large number of these creatures in an enclosed area without developing a distinctive odor in the house, yet the custodian of the animals seems oblivious to the assault of the pungent odor on the senses.

Herein lies the grand secret behind the workings of aromatherapy. We are, indeed, affected by the scents of the world around us. The aim of the aromatherapist is to capture the effects of these scents—both conscious and unconscious—and to blend them together in such a way that their effect is directed to a specific purpose. Within the pages of this book are many blends, both magickal and therapeutic, that have been designed to evoke given responses, remedying specific ailments or life situations. In the hands of the competent aromatherapist, the workings of nature—often subtle in their thrust—become the *gifts* of nature. In their highest applications, these gifts are for the benefit, the well-being, and the betterment of all of humankind.

Whether we utilize the art and science of aromatherapy for physical and mental wellness—as in its expression as a healing art—or to enhance our spirits and better the conditions of our lives as we undertake its magickal applications, we are beginning a journey of both knowledge and wonder. And to take the first steps, we need only follow our noses.

PART I

Body

The Principles of Aromatherapy

CHAPTER 1

History and Legend

The history of the use of scent is tied inseparably with the use of herbs and plant stuffs for sustenance. Before the rise of the first great civilization, the race of human animals had to resort to instinct for survival, much like their four-footed counterparts. One of the key senses tied to survival was scent.

We may not have senses as finely tuned as our primitive ancestors. We have less need to depend on smelling an approaching predator or recognizing the direction of food as its aroma is carried in the flight of a passing breeze, so we are slower alerting to the world about us. But we may suppose that our ancestors had highly honed sensitivities, for they needed them to ensure that they would survive another day.

It would make sense that in this time of heightened sensual stimulation the first roots of aromatherapy were planted. We can guess that as fire became a commonplace tool in the villages of the primitive tribes, cooking food gained in popularity. With the beginnings of the culinary arts, the first hints of aromatherapy must have also developed. People would have noticed that different plants gave off different aromas when put to the cooking fire. Likewise, plants produced varying effects on those who may have tended the flames. Perhaps one plant would make one drowsy, while another would make breathing easier, and still another would bring an unexplainable feeling of elation.

In these early times, these strange effects may have been attributed to the virtues of some local god or goddess, and the plant or herb made sacred to that particular deity. Hence, we may imagine the origin of the very first ritual incense, an offering by fire of a sacred plant to the honor of some popular divine power. But in the days of prehistory, we can only guess at the way things may have occurred.

What we do know is that the virtues of fragrance were not unknown in even the earliest civilizations. In Egypt, as early as 1500 B.C., the sacred scents of frankincense and myrrh were among the highly valued prizes brought home from trading expeditions to foreign lands. The distillation of substances into essential oils has been taking place at least since 400 B.C. in Egypt. In the ancient civilizations of Greece and Rome, fragrance was commonly used in both incense and essential oils.

The Orient was also no stranger to the virtues of aromatics. In China and Japan, fragrant incense was offered up for ritual use in praise of the gods as well as for the enhancement and special favor of those who gave themselves in marriage.

In India, the home of Tantric practice, fragrance is used liberally in the pursuit of spiritual and physical love. In fact, the ability to manufacture essential oils in this holy land may date back as far as 3000 B.C.!

The ancient Hebrews were known, as early as 1200 B.C., to use sacred incenses at their altars. The inhabitants of the lands of the prophet Mohammed discovered the process of alcohol distillation within the first century A.D., but had long used other forms of fragrance as well.

It is difficult to ascertain how much of the development of fragrant substances was independent and how much was inspired by trade with distant lands. However, if we may judge from the universality of the employment of scent, once a culture found the world of aroma, by whatever means, they held dearly to its use.

In fact, there are legends that arise from nearly every land that proclaim the sanctity of one fragrance or another. Many claim the origin of a plant or flower as the exclusive domain of a particular god, goddess, prophet, ruler, or hero. One of the most well-known legends is the tale of Narcissus. By the magick of the goddess Artemis, Narcissus fell in love with his own reflection in a pool of water. He found himself unable to turn away from the beautiful vision before him, yet he was unable to embrace the figure that he saw within the pool. In his frustration, he took his own life. As his blood soaked into the earth at the water's edge, up sprang the flower that still bears his name.

Also from the legendry of Greece comes the tale of the nymph Daphne. Pursued by the god Apollo, the maiden called on Gaia, goddess of the earth, to rescue her. The goddess obliged by turning her into a laurel tree. Unable to consummate his love for the nymph, Apollo was moved to tenderness at the sight of her new form. The laurel remains favored of and sacred to the Greek god.

In ancient Rome, the holly was a celebrated plant sacred to Saturn. It was abundant in the ancient winter festival of Saturnalia. As the season rises to claim the flora of the world for death, the green holly stands as the promise of rebirth, its color rich with life while the rest of the plant world has paled with the arrival of winter. The deep red berries are the color of blood, another hint that life continues on, even as the slumber of the earth through the bitter months seems to be the deep slumber of death. The sacred holly plant yet endures in our winter festivities to remind us of rebirth and renewal or, in the Christianized version, of the promise of renewed life through resurrection.

In India, there is a story told of the sacred lotus, the flower of Paradise. In order to obtain this holy blossom for his queen, an Indian hero named Bhima sets out on a dangerous journey. This sacred blossom is not easily sought or lightly plucked. It dwells in a sacred lake surrounded by a forest full of wild animals, evil spirits, and demons. Although Bhima was brave, in the end it was only through the safe passage granted by the ape-god Hanuman that the hero claimed his prize.

Moslem mythology credits the origin of certain plants to the prophet Mohammed. According to ancient lore, the rose first appeared at the sight where the prophet's sweat was spilled on the soil. The geranium also is credited to Mohammed. It is said that the first geranium blossom sprang from a hedge on which the holy man had hung his shirt to dry after washing it in a stream.

The tales of fragrant plants are endless. Some are little more than pleasant tales to delight the heart and stir the imagination. Others may hint at the application of some fragrances. The narcissus flower, for example, contains a narcotic oil. Just as Narcissus was gripped by the intoxicating vision of his own reflection in the water, the flower has an intoxicating effect upon the user. The rose, held sacred by the goddess of love, Aphrodite, is a common ingredient in many of the magickal blends famed for their properties of attraction.

No matter what the end application is of fragrant oils, theirs is a history and legendry that reaches back far into time. While it is true that an appreciation of aromatics developed early in the history of human civilization, it is difficult to ascertain exactly where lies the origin of fragrances for therapeutic purposes. There is evidence of very early use of aromatic herbs and incense blends being burned for purification, for a healthy spiritual state, and for proper preparation of the dead for the journey to the underworld, but the beginnings of aromatherapy as a healing art are more elusive. The earliest references to the art of the aromatherapist are either tied to the practice of magick or to the studies of the herbalist.

While fragrant substances have been coveted as prized treasures from the earliest days of prehistory, one of the earliest references to their application in the healing arts arises with the Black Death in Europe in the fourteenth century. A mixture of clove, cypress, pine, cedar, rosemary, and thyme was burned in the disease-ridden homes, hospitals, and even in the streets to cleanse the land of the plague. Although there is some cleansing and disinfecting virtue in this blend of aromatics, it is likely that its use was not totally divorced from magickal practice. Many of the applications of aromatics, though they may hint of therapeutic use, were not clearly recognizable as aromatherapy as it is practiced today. Modern aromatherapy, though it may be founded on the work of respected herbologists of the seventeenth and eighteenth centuries, is really a development from within the past hundred years.

The relative newness of the practice of healing with aromatics in no way compromises its value as a worthy alternative to orthodox medicine. While the development of the application is something out of modern innovation, the herbalists' work on which the methods of aromatherapy were founded has proven itself with time. In fact, in many respects, the art of herbal therapy may righteously claim to be the root of the whole of allopathic remedy as well as aromatherapy. Science has broken down the individual chemical components of abundant herbs and extracted or synthetically reproduced them to produce the pharmaceuticals that are now widely available.

The aromatherapist, not unlike the orthodox physician, adopts the virtue of the fragrance of natural substances, extracts it into oil or synthetically reproduces it, and uses it in the work of healing and health maintenance. In this respect, all of the healing arts and sciences—whether in the field of herbalism, the practice of allopathic healing, or the pursuit of aromatherapy—are tied inescapably with the gifts of nature.

CHAPTER 2

Science, Art, and Magick

The practice of aromatherapy exists in a plane that is made of the substance of two seemingly different worlds. As a system of healing the body, it is not unlike the pursuit of herbology. It is rooted in the healing arts of the earth, in the utilization of nature's gifts for the betterment of humankind. However, this ancient practice is not limited to the treatment of physical ills but can be used to improve the mental, and even the spiritual, condition as well. In this application, it is more closely aligned with the practice of natural magick. As a system, it is a complete approach to the human condition. It is neither strictly art nor strictly science. While aromatherapy has applications in physical healing, it does not fail to acknowledge the ailments of mind and spirit that are wont to plague human existence.

Although the lion's share of written material available on the use of scent to effect change addresses its application in the healing of the body, the effect of fragrances on the mind should not be understated. Many would agree that a healthy attitude in a patient is invaluable in effecting a speedy recovery from an ailment. Any treatment, whether medicinal, herbal, or aromatherapeutic, is most effective when offered to one who wants to recover.

The nature of aromatherapy is such that, when treating the physical structure, one cannot help but touch the mental facilities. It is the founding principle of healing with aromatic substances that the body responds differently to each unique scent. If this is true, can we suppose that the mind, which first receives the fragrant communication from the nasal passages, is immune to its effect? Not likely!

As with any other sensual impulse, scent is received and relayed to the mind for interpretation and response. We are more comfortable around some colors than others. Some adore the soft, cool feel of silk while others prefer the comforting warmth of wool. The steakhouses enjoy as brisk a business as the seafood restaurants. Music shops carry a variety of different types of musical expression to appease a rainbow of varying preferences.

The point is not that we each develop our own set of responses depending on individual life experiences but that we all do respond, in one way or another, to outside stimuli. This is the basis of aromatherapy.

The challenge of the aromatherapist is to take that natural capacity for reaction and direct it in specific ways for predetermined results. In light of the many differences between individuals, it is natural to question how we may standardize any such system dependent on anticipated response. We do this by cutting through experience and background to instinctive response. If we appeal to that part of us that yet remembers the scent of a food source that means survival or the scent of a predator that indicates danger, we can circumvent the conditioned responses and cut directly to the animal within. We awaken the beast that lives by instinct instead of wit, by necessity instead of preference, by survival instead of social doctrine.

On this base level, we respond in very like ways. Fear, confidence, pride, and love are not foreign to anyone. Desire, elation, satisfaction, and sorrow are common to all of us. The same instinct that was the facility of survival for our prehistoric ancestors remains with us in our capacity for emotion. And while allopathic medicine attempts to avoid arousing the inner self with tasteless, odorless pills, the aromatherapist seeks out these buried instincts to aid in the process of recovery.

This is the secret to where the scent therapist finds common ground in such a diverse menagerie of personality types. It is a difference in approach from much of the healing community, as it is the shared condition that is highlighted. And to touch the inner instinct is to raise a force that is more potent than the experiences of a single lifetime—it is to touch the facility that is interwoven with the spark of life itself. While experience is a product of how we choose to live our lives, and the inter-reaction with others with whom we share our daily existence, instinct is irretrievably bound up with the essence our lives. It is not how we live, but why we live.

There are so-called faith healers who ask simply that you believe. There are those who heal through hypnosis. These two apparently different approaches to healing are, in fact, equally supportive of the proposition that the mind can heal itself. And through the practice of aromatherapy, we must truly win over the mind before we can effectively create our desired changes in the body.

In this area, there are many principles to be acknowledged that cross over into some of the most ancient spiritual practices. The New Age concept of balancing the physical, mental, and spiritual selves is a cornerstone doctrine of many of the world's spiritual disciplines, though the way the concept is expressed may differ from one religious system to the next.

In the Orient, the concept of balancing yin and yang is rooted in the same type of thinking. These are the forces that embody the female and male forces that reside within each of us. They are the passive and the active, the mental and the physical, the mind and the body of the human makeup. It is when these complementing forces work in unison that the spiritual self is most healthy. In India or Tibet, this same sense of balance is sought through chakra work. The chakras are centers of consciousness located in a vertical line throughout the body. They correspond not only to different bodily functions such as reproduction, digestion, evacuation, circulation, respiration, and sensory recognition, but they also touch the base survival instincts that dwell within us all. They correspond to passion, hunger, the innate protective mechanisms of self-survival, and that unconscious, indescribable force that keeps us breathing in and out with no provocation from thought or reason. As in the case of yin and yang, when the chakras are in balance, they culminate in spiritual well-being.

After considering the major functions of the mental and spiritual facets of the human animal in maintaining and restoring a healthy existence, we might wonder if we can effect changes in the body directly or only through the vehicles of mind and spirit. Yet there do exist strictly physical responses to outside stimuli. A kettle of boiling water spilled on the skin may be interpreted in the mind as pain but there is also an immediate physical effect in the swelling and blistering of the affected area. Limbs may be broken, diseases contracted, and any number of ailments incurred. While it may be true that the mind has the ability to heal the body, and perhaps even stave off the maladies of physical existence, the body itself can be directly affected.

There are tales of those who overcome the physical world. There are the firewalkers of the Huna people in Hawaii and the Sufis with their mysterious ability to walk on glass or lay down upon the famed bed of nails. Most folks, however, have not been disciplined to overcome the physical world and are ready victims to the ills and mishaps of living a physical existence. The reality that most people can be affected by unfortunate physical circumstances, however, is also an indication that the condition of the body can be altered for the better as well.

The fact that there are people able to overcome physical ills illustrates the healing power that is available within the human mind if we can just stimulate it into action. Between affecting the mental facilities with fragrance and creating effects on the physical body with direct application, we have the foundation of the practice of aromatherapy.

Another aspect of aromatherapy that should not be neglected lies in the fact that, for the most part, we are dealing with natural extractions. Just as herbs or medical preparations drawn from the wealth of the earth's treasured resources can be used in healing applications, so are essential oils simply another form of the healing substances made available by nature. Whether ingested or applied externally, like many herbal remedies, or introduced directly into the bloodstream, like some of the miracle drugs of accepted medical practice, or applied topically or through inhalation, as in the practice of aromatherapy, we are ultimately dealing with the same source in our healing practices. All preparations— from the herbal tea to the antibiotic serum to the essential oil— take their origin from nature. They may go through different processes from natural state to end product, but they all originate from the gifts of nature.

Bringing Science, Art, and Magick Together

With so much common ground apparent within the spheres of the artistic, magickal, and scientific areas, and with nature at the root of each of the three disciplines, it is natural to wonder the exact difference between these three seemingly different areas of practice. In fact, it is merely a difference of approach. As hard as the purist may argue in defense of his or her own chosen discipline, each area crosses over into the others. The root of an approach of artistry, for example, may be considered the spark of inspiration that initiates action. While in aromatherapy, the faculty of inspired action is invaluable, even the formula that is borne of inspiration must be tested in accordance with the disciplines of the scientist in order to fulfill its purpose. The magickal aromatherapist, as well, must test the oil blend again and again in order to be assured of its effectiveness. No matter how determined the magician may be to see the magickal blend through to a predetermined result, the dedication of the pursuit will be to little avail if the blend itself is contrary to the purpose.

Then, there is the scientist. Armed with an analytical mind and a dedication to sound principles of experimentation, to a scientist the finished product must be a workable blend. It has been well thought out, thoroughly tested through repeated experiments, and its sound design will only be verified in its eventual application. The scientific approach alone seems to be structured as a truly disciplined factor. Yet the truth is that even the most disciplined scientist cannot hold off the influence of inspiration. Consider, for example, the invention of penicillin. There seems to be little scientific reason to utilize bread mold as a basis for a miracle drug. In fact, spoiled food has been at the root of many ailments that plague humanity. What possible basis would any right-thinking scientist have for believing that a substance that is at the root of suffering could be utilized to relieve it? Consider also some of the other medications that have been developed by the investigative hand of science. There are medications that use whale sperm, monkey hormones—any variety of strange substances. Although the development process may have remained within the rigorous boundaries of accepted scientific discipline, it must have been a spark of inspiration that was at the root of the experimentation that led to the many so-called miracle drugs of our time.

The truth is that the approaches of magick, art, and science are merely labels that serve little but the comfort of the individual practitioner. They are not the essence of the practice but the approach toward its process. At some point, each of the disciplines must acknowledge and utilize the benefits of the others. To achieve the highest degree of effectiveness, the scientific mind must learn to be open to the inspiration that moves the artist. The scientist may have to sometimes acknowledge that although there may be no sound scientific basis for a blend to be successful, it works simply because it does. Perhaps it is because it was borne of inspiration or maybe it is inexplicable because its functioning is magickal. The artist must use the instinctive inspiration that drives his or her being as a basis for formulation of a blend, yet must borrow the disciplines of the scientist to ensure that it is effective. Even the magician cannot escape the trappings of the other two practitioners. If a formula is ineffective, no matter how strong the magician's drive might be to see the success of a magickal operation, the ineffective blend will do little more than to throw obstacles in the path of the ultimate success of the magickal intention.

In essence, the three apparent disciplines of Art, Magick, and Science in the practice of aromatherapy are largely illusions. The differences between the way that individual practitioners think and feel will color their approach to aromatherapy. It will dictate the manner in which any one individual may function best, or most comfortably. In truth, the only acceptable practice of scent working is one that is effective. Whether the individual practitioner chooses to attribute the success of the blends that emerge from aromatherapy to any or all of these seemingly opposed disciplines is moot; in fact, all three will have to be utilized to some degree if their practice is workable. In your own pursuit of the creation of oil blends, you may consider yourself what you wish—artist, magician, or scientist. The only true measure of the practice is this: Does your created scent find its resting place in successful application? For only then does one become a true aromatherapist.

CHAPTER 3

*A*romatic Sense

Considerations in Aromatherapy

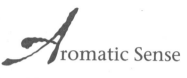

Consider the homecoming of a traveler, navigating
the way through field and wood, headed toward
the comfort of familiar surroundings and the
welcoming embrace of loved ones. As
the road draws to an end,
our traveler may arrive
on the edge of a
meadow that lies just
outside the familiar
family home. The soft
scent of heather fills the
nostrils and elates the heart

with the certain knowledge that home is near. As the field fades in the distance by a steady gait, the aroma of spaghetti and Grandpa's old world sauce fills the air. As the scent surrounds our traveler, the senses of comfort and well-being as well as the feelings of warmth and love swell up in the heart. This is the essence of the magick of scent.

While we readily understand the use of fragrance as an extension of herbal healing, the mental and spiritual effect of scents upon the human condition may seem a bit more elusive. But this elusive faculty is imperative to deriving the maximum benefit from aromatherapy. We have all seen, heard, or read about the patient who stops responding to treatment simply because he or she has lost the will to live. When dealing in the healing arts, we cannot divorce the act of healing the body from that of nurturing the mind and spirit. We cannot divorce the science or the art from the magick. They are all interrelated and interdependent. So while we may address the different applications of fragrance separately, we cannot view them as separate practices. They not only overlap but, in the hands of a competent scent mixologist, will enhance each other.

The actual functioning of a scent may vary in the way it works from one essential to another. Some scents create effects in their own right, while others function by association. Orange, for example, may create a mood of elation to relieve melancholy. This effect is inherent in the fragrance itself. Sandalwood, on the other hand, may be employed as something of an aphrodisiac. This effect is created, not by the fragrance in its own right, but by association. Its scent is not unlike that of a human sexual scent, or pheromone, being like that of alpha androsterole and, as such, has effects that parallel nature's own scent of arousal.

Like these specific examples, there are associated values that are inherent within each fragrance. These are the virtues that have been pursued for centuries by the perfumer, the healer, the magician, and in our own age, the practicing aromatherapist.

Natural versus Synthetic Oils

The medium we use will be that of essential oils, for these are the most potent and easily usable form of nature's aromas. While some students of aromatherapy restrict their practice to natural fragrances, others make use of synthetic substitutes too. Because the art is based on response to scent, it must be questioned whether it truly makes a difference whether that aroma is extracted from nature or earnestly replicated in the laboratory. If the difference is undetectable, will the resulting effect not be the same, as well?

Another argument in defense of the employment of synthetic scents is on a practical level. Because of the difficulty of extracting certain oils or the rarity of the host plant in nature, the cost of the end product can be prohibitive. There is an oil that is derived from a lily that grows only in one particular region in France. The cost of the natural essential oil would run into the thousands of dollars per ounce. Meanwhile, a good synthetic of this same scent can be purchased for well under a hundred dollars for an entire pound.

While it might be argued that the natural essence would have a higher level of effectiveness, this is really a moot point. Because the synthetic has a proven track record, it ought not be discounted as a valid alternative to the unavailable and cost-prohibitive natural product. In my own practice, I use the readily available naturals but will not undervalue the virtues of a good synthetic essence when the natural oil is not readily available or priced too dearly.

Irritant Oils

Among the many considerations to be noted before going full steam into the practice of aromatherapy is that of the oils themselves. Certain oils are irritants and may have an ill effect in external application, or even in use as inhalants. The most pronounced of these are noted as irritants in the text by the use of the exclamation mark (!). However, it is a caution well heeded to acknowledge that, when dealing with different people, they may carry different sensitivities with them. This includes, but is not limited to, allergies. For example, there was one family I worked with who had an apparent inherited sensitivity to canola oil. Usually considered a harmless oil, in the case of this family the negative effects created in using this oil could far outweigh any benefits that might have been realized. For the responsible worker of fragrance, then, the bottom line is to know who you are working with as well as the properties of the oil blends you employ.

Traditional Approaches

There are two primary areas to be addressed in using fragrance as a medium for effecting changes in the human condition. We must develop some criteria for the mixing of specific scents in blended oils and we must arrange some way of utilizing the prepared oil blends.

First, it should be remembered that the roots of aromatherapy lie far in the past. Like many of the ancient arts, they are designed with regard to the belief systems that were common in ages past. And in the specific case of scent therapy, its background is shared in many ways with the ancient herbalist.

One of the earliest published recognized voices of authority in the field of herbalism was that of Nicholas Culpeper. In *Culpeper's Complete Herbal and English Physician*, originally published in 1826, Mr. Culpeper gives us the foundation of his system of arriving at the proper combination of ingredients to formulate specific remedies. The earliest systems of science were a delightful mixture of the fruits of new discovery within the framework of the ancient arts of healing. Even within the descriptive passages included on the title pages, Culpeper tells his readers that this offering includes descriptions of several hundred herbs along with "a display of their medicinal and occult properties."

Herbology, like its related practice of aromatherapy, has never been totally isolated from its roots in the ancient religio-occult studies of our ancestors. In reviewing some of Culpeper's entries on specific herbs, it becomes evident that he was keenly aware of the astrological and elemental virtues of each plant he culled from the fields and mountains, and that these properties dictated their application as components in healing remedies.

In his written selection on lavender, Culpeper notes

> Being an inhabitant almost in every garden, it is so well known, that it needeth no description. . . . Mercury owns the herb, and it carries its effects very potently. . . . The chemical oil drawn from lavender, usually called oil of spike, is of so fierce and piercing a quality, that it is cautiously to be used, some few drops being sufficient, to be given with other things either for inward or outward griefs.

Similarly, in his selection on lily of the valley, the properties of the plant are listed as "under the dominion of Mercury, and therefore strengthens the brain, recruits a weak memory, and makes it strong again." Honeysuckle is given as a "hot martial plant in the celestial sign of Cancer. . . . The oil made by infusion of the flowers is accounted healing and warming, and good for the cramp and convulsion of the nerves."

In the summary passages of his herbal, Nicholas Culpeper states that the included herbs are virtuous as healing remedies, "and the plain reason thereof is this, because they are governed, made rich, preserved, and are every way made proper and fit to heal the body of man . . . by the celestial ministers of Heaven." Although we do not turn a deaf ear to whatever advances may be made by modern researchers to our art, its foundation and its creation lie in the arcane knowledge of the old astrologers and alchemists. In fact, the contribution of science often is most valuable in defining why the systems of ancient healing work. The fact that these methods have survived through countless centuries is evidence enough that they work, but it is often helpful to couple the effectiveness of a particular remedy with knowledge of its physiological effects. In this way we can reap the benefits of both worlds, the old and the new. Hopefully, the marriage of the two spheres of working will result in an increased level of effectiveness in both the fields of medicine and the natural healing arts.

Applications of Aromatherapy

In addressing the traditional approach to aromatherapy, it is important to investigate the application or method of employment of the fragrant mediums. These are, to some extent, dependent on the situation to be remedied, and must take into account the particular situation and, at times, the particular recipient of the application. We must keep in mind that each person is born with varying sensitivities, and may respond better to one method of application than another.

It also must be considered to which purpose an aromatic mixture is to be directed. While there are those who enter into the field of aromatherapy strictly for its benefits in physical healing, others pursue the magickal aspects of the art and direct their efforts to improving the human condition as well as the state of the body and mind. That being said, there are general applications that are common to both facets of aromatherapy: inhalation and external application.

Inhalation

Inhalation is the more widely used method of delivering scent. One of the earliest uses of herbs in their natural state, in fact, was through inhalation therapy in a system called "smoking." The herb was burned and the fumes inhaled by the ailing individual to effect relief from whatever malady was being treated. It is easy to see the direct relation of this method of treatment to the burning of incense in the temples of ancient civilization, one of the earliest methods of magickal aromatherapy. Although essential oils have become the central medium of aromatherapy practice, the employment of aromatic herbs in their natural state should not be forgotten. It remains a viable form of utilizing the properties of fragrance.

Today, there are many other alternative methods to accomplishing inhalation therapy. There are oil diffusers available that can fill a room with fragrance. There are potpourri cookers widely available (a modification of the smoking method). Of course thuribles, or incense burners, are also in no shortage of supply. Light rings, vaporizers, direct and indirect inhalation—the available equipment and the methods are many. These will be addressed in more than a conceptual manner as we delve into the actual physical workings of the aromatherapist's art. At this point, what is important to recognize is that inhalation methods account for a great bulk of the applications of aromatherapy.

External Application

External application is also employed in both the healing and the magickal facets of aromatherapy. There is sometimes a preference in the specific area of the body to which an essential oil is applied. In chakra work, it may seem advantageous to pointedly include or exclude certain traditional chakra centers, depending on the condition to be remedied. This can be true whether it is a magickal or healing endeavor that is being undertaken. In treating certain ailments of the body, topical dressings may be employed in only the affected areas. Again, this may depend on the nature of the specific problem being addressed. Like the use of fragrance in inhalation, there is more than one method of applying a remedy externally.

This may be accomplished through the use of perfumed oils and waters, through fragrant baths, in combination with massage therapy or, in magickal use, the aromatic substance may be applied to a separate object that is representative of the individual on whose condition the change is to be enacted.

Though there have been a significant number of advances in how fragrances may be administered to effect change, the basic methods remain as they have for centuries. Though we use the improvements of modern science and manufacturing, we have not altered the facilities employed by the ancient ancestors of the modern aromatherapists. We have only developed some alternatives in how we might deliver the virtue of fragrance for the betterment of the human condition.

Aromatic Sense

It cannot be stressed enough how the approach to aromatherapy is all important. Whether there is a leaning toward the healing applications of the art or to the magickal aspects, or to both, the approach may well determine the ultimate success or failure of the endeavor.

Many practicing aromatherapists work by instinct alone. For many, with a background of extensive study, research, and experimentation, the instincts can take over and do an admirable job of guiding the practice of the art. In watching the seasoned experts work, it is fascinating to see the overwhelming light of creativity and inspiration that go into the final production of an essential oil blend. It becomes clearly understandable why this ancient practice, while full of the trappings of the scientific pursuits, remains very much an art form, as well.

Those, however, who are new to the ways of fragrance blending may want to do things more by the book. It is conceivable that, somewhere beneath the layers of learned, conditioned behavior, we all have the capacity to set free our instinctive knowledge and let it guide our steps to effective and practical applications of aromatherapy. For the beginning student of fragrance working, however, it is far more advisable to base the decisions as to what ingredients belong in a particular oil blend on sound knowledge gleaned from sincere study. Let instincts develop as they may in accordance with natural individual growth. After generations of ignoring instinctual knowledge as a matter of social conditioning, one could hardly expect to become an expert overnight. Don't rush the process!

The formulae included in this volume include many of the more traditional blends as well as some of the newer designs. The old traditional combinations may be considered tried and true. They have been utilized for many years throughout their host cultures and any other societies that may have adapted them into their own systems of healing and magick. Also included are many of the newer developments. These have been designed and produced for optimum effectiveness for use in their given purpose.

Even armed with these most powerful proven blends, however, the approach to the art of aromatherapy must be rational. While we share a universal existence as a people, we are also endowed—especially with the advent of higher communication and travel—with our own set of experiences and response stimuli. As we deal with individuals in aromatherapy (or any art) we must always safeguard against losing the integrity of the lone client in the shared experiences of the masses.

We live our lives as individuals, perhaps coming together in many different kinds of bonds but still as individuals in our own right. As individuals it is possible, and even likely, that one client may not respond in a textbook manner to a certain fragrance or fragrant blend. Rather, one person's response may be colored by personal experience.

Though many may think of aromatherapy as a science, it should never be characterized by the strict disciplines of the more orthodox scientific processes but should be left flexible. After all, we utilize the virtues of the art of aromatherapy for the betterment of the individual. We can hardly hope to accomplish this lofty undertaking by giving credence to the universal truths of the art and ignoring the client. We must remain flexible and sensitive if our resulting journey into aromatherapy is to be effective.

This is the essence of what we might call "aromatic sense." Because aromatherapy is steeped in both science and art, and because we must adhere to principles of both universal and individual response to scent, the practice demands a special kind of discipline of its own. It is a balancing of virtues that make it work. The knowledge, study, and experimentation facilities are there, just as might be found in a chemistry lab. Amounts of individual components of an oil blend are exacting, often measured in drops. Yet an open mind and sensitive nature are also essential for the optimal practice of aromatherapy. Because we deal with individuals and create effects on people's physical, mental, and spiritual conditions, we cannot approach the design of a blend with a purely black and white, action and reaction, stimulus and response, dry, scientific attitude. Our working must be tempered with a sensitivity to the needs and responses of the individual and, above all, laced with compassion.

In offering a complete presentation of the workings of aromatherapy, perhaps we should expand our understanding of "psychological" to include all that is non-physical. It is important to note that scent can have a significant effect on the emotional and the spiritual as well as the strictly mental facilities of humankind.

Aromatic substances—herbs, plants, and essential oils—work on the non-physical self via different avenues. The deepest, most ingrained level of response is that of instinct. Nature has gifted all animals, humans and other species, with an instinct for survival. One of the keys to unleash this natural function is scent. Whether survival translates as the continuation of the individual life or the propagation of the race, there is a specific aroma-response system at work that serves as a catalyst to awaken the inborn facility. During the courting or arousal stages of sexual activity, hormones (in this case, pheromones) are secreted to accompany the ritual. A reaction to the scent of the natural aromas helps build the emotional state to a crescendo and the physical act of sexual congress to consummation. Essential oil blends can be produced to emulate the fragrance of natural hormones. On a therapeutic level, such remedies can be used to minister to frigidity and impotence. On a magickal level, we have the development of the well-known love oils or love potions that enrich the folklore and folk practices of many cultures throughout the world.

Again, if we can refer to the primitive beast for our knowledge, there is another faculty that is intimately tied with the instinct for survival. The animal is alerted to the approach of impending danger. If a predator nears, it is the scent of the predator that may first alert the animal to the situation. To capture this scent and expose it to the animal, it would set the animal on edge. Considering this in a therapeutic application, the scent of danger might well be a cure for apathy or awaken the importance of individual worth in one suffering from low self-esteem. It could be enlisted to tone down conceit or to interject a sober note to one who is over the edge. It could give a touch of reality to those who are prone to living in fantasy. Overall, enlisting the reaction to scents of danger would tend to lend a sobering, stabilizing force to the psyche.

While these reactions to scent are universal and very ingrained in the two-legged and four-legged beasts, as well as the creatures of water and air, there are yet other response facilities that can be tapped in the case of the human animal. While many of these are commonly shared, some are exclusive to a certain individual or group of individuals. These are the responses that are dictated by experience rather than by natural instinct.

Most flower scents evoke pleasant memories. There may be the treasured memories of youth—times spent with friends and lovers in fields of wildflowers or the cultured gardens of a favorite quiet place. The smell of hickory may be reminiscent of barbecues with friends and family. Rosemary or sage may evoke thoughts of kitchen times. The spicy fullness of Grandma's homemade spaghetti sauce may also bring the certain feeling that we are loved and secured against all the world's ills.

On the converse side, scent can bring back dreaded times of the past. The fragrance of wildflowers, while it is likely to be pleasing to most, could have a markedly different effect on one who was lost in such a field as a child. Where many of us would find love and friendship carried with the fragrance, this individual might be carried to fear and loneliness. The hickory scent that reminds many of us of wonder- ful times spent with beloved family members may represent the outdoor flame that was ignited to cook a favorite pet rabbit when the family's need overtook the special bond of love that a child knew with the furry friend. The spices that remind us of our kindly grandmother may well be the same scent that evokes visions of a grandmother who was not so kindly and who did not make her grandchildren feel secure and loved.

So it is with the art of aromatherapy. Whether directed toward therapeutic or magickal purposes, it should be remembered that, in addition to the inborn facilities of response to scent, the human animal has a whole world of individual experiences that will affect response to aroma. Herein lies one of the greatest cautions—and the greatest responsibilities—of the aromatherapist: know your patient! While it is possible to suggest the probable response to a given fragrance for the general masses, when applying the principles of aromatherapy we are not dealing with the masses but with specific individuals. Therefore, we must be ready to monitor response to a remedy every step of the way, and willing to alter our formulas to custom-suit them to the individual. Although the standard formulas may prove very effective for some, not everyone will be positively responsive to the over-the-counter brand of therapy. In fact, in some, the traditional blends could prove counterproductive.

Humankind is a living, thinking, feeling race of being. While we can capture and control certain responses for the betterment of the individual, aromatherapy is an uncertain science in that the practitioner must be always aware and adaptable. While yellow and blue will always make green on the canvas of the artist, it is the task of the painter to be certain that it is the right shade of green for the particular scene. Likewise, it is the responsibility of the fragrance artist to monitor and ascertain that a particular blend is properly fitting to the given situation. Although undeniably artistic in their thrust, both painter and aromatherapist are motivated by the end result. It matters little how pretty or how fragrant the medium but how it affects the overall picture—the whole individual.

CHAPTER 4

Responsible Aromatherapy and Magickal Ethics

*E*ach time we apply the ancient healing and
magickal arts we are creating changes in the
lives of our clients and often in the lives of those
individuals around them. Our entire
existence in this world is
made up of a series of
contacts with others.
We laugh together, play
together, share loves,
sorrows, joys, and
tears, and unveil the
deepest secrets of our
souls, one to the other.

Each blend that emerges from the table of the aromatherapist must carry with it the responsibility of the effects that it will bring to people's lives.

In its healing applications, this is obviously true. Just as we may help someone to recuperate from an ailment or relieve pain and suffering, our work could also function to worsen the condition of the one we seek to help. Just as different individuals may have a negative reaction to certain medications, so may there be similar unfavorable responses to specific scents. There may be allergic reactions to specific essential oil ingredients to consider. It is the responsibility of the practicing aromatherapist to not only blend the correct ingredients for the particular condition that is to be remedied but the correct ingredients for the particular individual as well.

There are certain oils that are irritant oils. While there may be some people who have little or no negative reaction to these oils, others may suffer considerable discomfort when in contact with these scents through breathing their aromas or through physical contact with the skin. Likewise, there are specific oils that are almost universally accommodating. These are the carrier oils. Sometimes, these user-friendly oils may be used to dilute the effect of an otherwise irritating essential oil. In the appendix, there are lists of both these essential oil types. But a word of caution—do not ignore the individual response factor! One of the most unusual situations I have encountered so far in the application of aromatherapy has been the uncovering of an allergic reaction to a carrier oil. Out of three family members treated, the mother and one daughter had the exact same allergic response to the supposedly universally acceptable oil. The responsible aromatherapist deals with the foundation principles of the art but does not close his or her eyes to the real life people for which the art is plied. Braced with the knowledge of the ancient wisdom of aromatherapy, the fragrance artisan also has eyes wide open toward the effects created through the practice as they unfold.

On the magickal side of aromatherapy, there are additional complications in responsible working. While involved in therapeutic use, there is little question of ethics. To relieve an ailment or ease the suffering of a fellow human being—how can there be a question as to the virtue of the act? In the magickal application, however, there are many questions that may arise. Remember that when an effect is created on one individual, it also exerts an influence on those directly and indirectly involved with that individual. The one who is responsible for effecting this change should also be willing to stand up for the thrust of any backlash that may occur from it.

The possible solutions are few. Either do not pursue the magickal side of fragrance arts or else enter into it in a responsible manner. There are many ways to define the righteousness of a magickal undertaking. One of the most simple is one that was given to me through my own studies in the magickal arts. Before making a decision to pursue a magickal undertaking, the question must be addressed whether or not this is an operation that is good for everyone it touches. To determine this, use the following three-circle system of magickal responsibility.

The Three-Circle System

Before undertaking any magickal working, write down the names of those who are directly involved. If this undertaking is unquestionably to the greatest benefit of all those listed, draw a circle around the names. Next, consider those who might be once removed from the immediate cast of players. Is this act to the greater benefit of these people—the brothers, sisters, parents, and closest friends? If you can honestly see benefit, draw another circle around this cast of characters once removed. Finally, take the analysis out to another level. Consider the grocer, the teacher, the clergy, the neighborhood poet, and the village idiot. Will the completion of this magickal act be favorable in their lives? If so, then draw a third circle. If you can get through three circles, then what you are about to do is an act of righteous goodness and worthy of the effort. If you cannot get through three circles, or don't know enough about the situation to answer whether this is a positive change or not, then it is an ill-advised action. It is wise to not enter into it or at least to put it aside until you learn more about the situation.

For another example of this three-circle system in action, assume that you are about to take on a love rite. Draw three concentric circles. In the center, place the names of the two who will be bonded together, say Mary and Roger. Is this something that will impact Mary in a positive manner? How about Roger? If the undertaking is something that will be a positive change for both people involved, you've passed the first level of responsibility. Congratulations! Now, on to the next level.

In the second circle, write the names of those in the immediate sphere of the two lovers. How will this action affect Mary's mother, her brother, her pet tarantula? Well, Mary's mother adores Roger, and her brother has already asked to be the best man should they marry. The tarantula seems as comfortable with Roger as he does with Mary. Looks good. So what about the other side? How will this union affect the aunt and uncle that raised Roger? What about Roger's sister? What about Roger's . . . wife?! Uh-oh! See the need for responsible action?

Let's take it to another level. Suppose there is no wife, and everyone in the immediate lives of the would-be lovers are all for their union. What about Mary's mother's bridge club? What about her brother's fiancée? What about Roger's Uncle's fishing buddies?

What about his sister's best friend? A little obtuse? Perhaps—but only if it is possible to get through all three levels of investigation can you enter into the magickal rites honorably. If there is a problem, maybe this undertaking is not such a good idea. If you can't even get to the third level, perhaps you don't know enough about the situation to even consider magickal process. There is a fine line between help and meddling.

Whatever the approach to a magickal endeavor, having observed the proper ceremony to ensure the responsibility of the operation and chosen a method of working, there are many areas to be pursued in regard to the magickal effect of the medium of aromas. In addition to their physical attributes, essential oils also have magickal properties that should be observed for maximum effectiveness in the magickal arena. These should be learned as well as the physical properties, and are delineated further in the chapters that follow.

PART II

Mind

The Practice of Aromatherapy

CHAPTER 5

The Oils

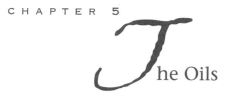

Essential oil is manufactured from the oil contained within a plant or flower, the essence of the entity. In order for it to be used by the aromatherapist, it must first be extracted from its host. There are numerous ways to accomplish this. Some of these methods are preferred for the quality of the yield. Because of the need to employ costly and complicated equipment in certain methods of extraction, they are resigned to the laboratories of commercial enterprises. Other methods are more conducive to kitchen chemistry.

One caution on entering into a decision as to which process would be best suited to an individual's needs and abilities would be to develop an awareness of the quality level of the end product. In certain instances, it may be nearly impossible to manufacture an essential oil at home that could even begin to approach the same quality standards of what may be purchased from a commercial concern. For example, it is nearly impossible to get a quality product through home manufacturing methods with many woods and resins. The final selection of oils that is employed in practice may actually include some representatives of both commercial and home manufacture.

Depending on the method of extraction used, there may be a lesser or greater percentage of actual plant essence in the finished product. While many companies label their products as essential oils, in truth, they contain essential oils in varying amounts. A distillation process, for instance, may result in a pure oil extract, while a heating process extracts the essence into a non-scented or low-scented carrier oil, diluting the end product. The system employed to obtain the essence from its natural state may be a factor in determining how potent an oil is and how aromatic it is for application.

Some varieties of plants contain essence in only very tiny amounts. One of these is a French variety of lily of the valley known as muguet. Large quantities of the host plant must be harvested in order to extract enough essential oil with which to work. In consideration of cost, time, and labor as well as the preservation of the natural environment, there are many synthetic oils that are produced to replace the natural essential product. These are made from substituted raw materials designed to emulate the fragrance of the natural essential oil. The original civet oil, for example, was first produced from the musk glands of cats in ancient Egypt. It is now offered as a synthetic blend in a humanitarian gesture to its feline hosts.

Methods of Extraction

As to the manufacture of essential oils, there are at least five common methods that may be employed to obtain the final product. These are enfleurage, maceration, evaporation, expression, and distillation. Although there are some peculiar variations of these, in general these are the basic ways in which to extract essential oils from nature.

Enfleurage

Enfleurage has been in use since ancient times. One of the attractions of this method is the romanticism of revisiting the ways of the past, and also that it requires no fancy equipment and is suitable for the home production of fragrant oils. The raw flowers or herbs are soaked in a host or carrier oil, and the essence is absorbed by the liquid. After a couple of days, the plant matter is removed and replaced by fresh material. This process is repeated until the remaining oil is of the scent potency desired.

Originally, animal fat may have been used in the process of enfleurage. However, for use in aromatherapy, many disdain the use of animal byproducts. The oil that is now normally used for extraction is one with little scent of its own. Some good candidates are sesame, sunflower, calendula, or almond (unlike the common synthetics that are designed to capture the fragrance of the plant, true almond oil actually has very little scent).

Maceration

Maceration is a method similar to enfleurage and may be nearly as dated in its employment. The major difference between the two systems is that, in maceration, the plant material is crushed before being immersed in oil to extract its essence. As in the prior method, after a few days, the herb or flower is strained out of the solution and replaced with freshly crushed leaves or blossoms. This process is repeated until the desired scent potency is reached.

One method of speeding the process of extraction is the introduction of heat. A popular way to accomplish this is to leave the vessel of soaking herbs in the sun, similar to the brewing of sun tea. Culpeper suggests that an appropriate cooking time is about a fortnight, or two weeks, depending on the season and directness of the sun's rays.

Evaporation

A third method of manufacturing essential oil products is through evaporation. In this method, solvents are employed for the extraction of the fragrant essence. This is a multi-step process. The plant is sealed up in a container with a solvent such as benzene. The essence is drawn into the solvent. The accomplishment of this first procedure is easily recognized by the strong aroma adopted by the solvent. Often, the plant material will also become limp and faded. Its color is often drawn out along with its fragrance. After this step is complete, the solvent solution is heated. One of the characteristics of solvents is that they have a low boiling point. As the solvent boils away, the plant essence that was drawn into it remains. This can be added to a low-scent oil to make a usable essential oil or it may be mixed with alcohol to make a tincture of the essence.

Expression

Expression is employed primarily in commercial development of essential oils. This is accomplished through cold pressing the plant materials in order to squeeze out the essence from the host. Because a great deal of pressure is required to arrive at the end product, this is a method that is best left to the factories, with their advanced and often costly machinery. A hand press cannot arrive at the same quality product that is possible through commercial development.

Distillation

Another ancient system for manufacturing essential oils is distillation. While this does require some equipment, it is not unlike the homemade stills that have speckled the hill country for generations, producing moonshine. The plants or flowers are either boiled or steamed in a closed cooker that culminates in a thin tube. As the pressure in the unit heightens, the extracted oil will rise to the top of the boiling water. It is then forced through the tube and collected by a waiting container as it drips out.

*I*ntroduction to Individual Oils

There are many different oils available through commercial purchase and home manufacture. Different practitioners of the fragrance arts may favor varying scents in different applications. Some are more widely used for healing applications, and some are more commonly employed in magickal pursuits. In any case, it should be remembered that there is more than one way to arrive at the desired results. And while there are certain oils that have been discovered to function well for specific purposes, when we combine fragrances for a specific goal, there is a lot of room for the individual aromatherapist's expression of knowledge and creativity. By utilizing varying amounts of different scents, a skillful aromatherapist may emphasize one quality or another in the final blend. It is in this facility that the science of aromatherapy retains its integrity as an art.

The oils included in this writing are by no means the full complement of available essentials. In fact, they are but a sampling of the products that may be found in my own selection of oils. However, they do represent a solid cross-section of the many products that may be used in aromatherapy.

In the tables that follow, each of the listed oils includes associations to gender, planetary affiliation, and elemental characteristics. While these attributes are more elaborately addressed in chapter 9, it may be important to at least offer some foundational understanding of the included associated influences in the oils presented below. The gender associations are simple male and female; in a very broad sense, these are active and passive, conscious and subconscious. They are the yin and yang of Oriental understanding. Together they create a balance, but in their separate roles they can be utilized in a specific approach to a specific purpose. The planetary influences are akin to the precedent set by Nicholas Culpeper in his presentation of herbal remedies. Each of the planets and astrological signs has an influence of its own. Each essential oil is aligned with one or more of these influences. From these associations, we can gain some valuable insight as far as the use of each of the essentials is concerned. By blending different influences, we arrive at an unlimited number of possibilities of uses for essential oils. These associations will serve as a guidebook in the blending of essential oils to specific purposes and optimum effectiveness.

One point that may be made before addressing the individual oils is that there is some variance between experts in regard to planetary or elemental associations. There is a legitimate reason for this sort of confusion. First, some plants have different variations. While some may be attuned to one influence, other variations of the same plant may be more representative of other associations. A prime example of this would be jasmine. While many aromatherapists view jasmine as a masculine fragrance representative of Jupiter, the night-blooming jasmine may be more akin to lunar influence and feminine in nature. Unfortunately, while some essential oils are very specific as to the particular plant variation from which they are derived, many are not. Another possible explanation of this apparent inconsistency is in application. While a specific oil may have certain characteristics as a lone remedy, in combination with other fragrances it may act in slightly different ways. My own interpretation of this is that while each scent has its primary characteristics, they each also carry a secondary persona, or undertone value. For this reason, wherever possible, a secondary planetary and elemental influence is noted in each of the oil delineations.

! Irritant oils have been marked with the inclusion of an
• exclamation point (!) after the oil name.

Amber

Description	A hard, translucent yellow, orange, or brown resin often used for jewelry. This natural substance does not occur in oil form, nor can a true essential oil be pressed from the natural resin. The amber oils generally available are composed of other natural oils, often with some crushed amber added.
Planetary Influence	Jupiter
Secondary Planet	Moon (especially in crescent phase)
Elemental Association	Earth
Secondary Element	Water
Zodiac Influence	Libra
Mental/Emotional Effects	Stability, self-confidence
Healing Properties	General wellness, physical maintenance
Magickal Properties	Restoration, settling, end to turmoil, peace

Ambergris

Description	True ambergris is a gray waxy substance that is produced naturally by sperm whales. The cost of producing an essential oil from the actual source would be prohibitive and counter to the balance of nature. Most ambergris oil, therefore, is synthetic.
Planetary Influence	Venus
Secondary Planet	Mars
Elemental Association	Water
Secondary Element	Fire
Zodiac Influence	Taurus
Mental/Emotional Effects	An awakener, sparks interest, arouses curiosity, dispels apathy

Healing Properties	Tonic, stimulant, a booster added to therapeutic blends when subject is slow to respond
Magickal Properties	Arouses emotion, opens the door to affairs of the heart

Apple

Description	Oil may be pressed from the blossoms of the tree or derived from the fruit, or the skin of the fruit, itself. Some traders carry specifically separate scents for apple and apple blossom. Others use a combination of the fruit and flower scents.
Planetary Influence	Neptune
Secondary Planet	Venus
Elemental Association	Water
Secondary Element	Air
Zodiac Influence	Libra
Mental/Emotional Effects	Antidepressant, helps alleviate antisocial behavior, promotes self-confidence
Healing Properties	Stimulant, general well-being, tonic, helps allay hypochondria
Magickal Properties	Instills joy, happiness, promotes friendship, success

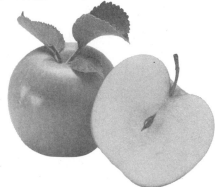

Bay

Description	The bay leaf is a common staple in the kitchen. This is the same plant that is used for essential oil, and comes from the laurel tree. In history, we also remember the bay laurel as the badge of honor presented to conquering heroes and victorious artists, athletes, and soldiers in ancient Greece.
Planetary Influence	Sun
Secondary Planet	Jupiter
Elemental Association	Fire
Secondary Element	Earth
Zodiac Influence	Aries, Leo
Mental/Emotional Effects	Dispels confusion, encourages clarity of thought
Healing Properties	Tonic, stimulant, disinfectant
Magickal Properties	Insight, clarity, awareness, peace, inspiration, also attracts money

Bergamot (!)

Description	The essential oil is extracted from the fruit of the bergamot tree, which is cultivated in Italy. It is a citrus family member.
Planetary Influence	Sun
Secondary Planet	Jupiter
Elemental Association	Fire
Secondary Element	Air
Zodiac Influence	Sagittarius
Mental/Emotional Effects	Eases grief, enhances self-image, antidepressant

Healing Properties	Aids digestion, antispasmodic, carminative, stimulant, antidepressant, antiseptic, sedative, expectorant, vulnerary
Magickal Properties	Happiness, peace, energy, may be used to enhance the effect of other oils or oil blends

Benzoin

Description	Also known as gum benjamin, benzoin is one of the oldest traditional ingredients of incense. It comes from the styrax tree and is commonly gathered in the island countries of Java, Thailand, and Sumatra.
Planetary Influence	Sun
Secondary Planet	Mercury
Elemental Association	Fire
Secondary Element	Air
Zodiac Influence	Aries, Gemini
Mental/Emotional Effects	Relieves guilt, builds sense of self-acceptance and trust
Healing Properties	Antiseptic, carminative, diuretic, expectorant, sedative, vulnerary
Magickal Properties	Boosts sensuality, promotes communication. Especially good for use in rituals that bring peace of mind. Well known as an ancient oil of offering.

Camphor (!)

Description Camphor originates from evergreen trees native to the Orient. The essence develops throughout the body of the tree but requires about a half century for its formation. Only very old trees are used for the production of this aromatic.

Planetary Influence Moon

Secondary Planet Saturn

Elemental Association Water

Secondary Element Earth

Zodiac Influence Cancer

Mental/Emotional Effects Calming, relieves shock, soothes anxiety, eases irritability, stimulates memory

Healing Properties Analgesic, antidepressant, antiseptic, antispasmodic, carminative, diuretic, hypertensive, laxative, sedative, vulnerary. Camphor also has some application as a stimulant—to kick start the digestive and respiratory systems and pick up the heart rate.

Magickal Properties Awakens past life memories, stimulates psychic awareness, may also be used as a power oil

Carnation

Description Often seen in the lapel of the awkward but dashing tuxedoed teen on prom night, this familiar scent is traceable in its oil form to ancient Greece. Its common nature makes it a popular and very affordable essential.

Planetary Influence Venus

Secondary Planet Sun

Elemental Association	Air
Secondary Element	Fire
Zodiac Influence	Aries, Libra
Mental/Emotional Effects	Enhances positive outlook, arouses will and determination
Healing Properties	General health, tonic, stimulant
Magickal Properties	Love, health, energy, luck

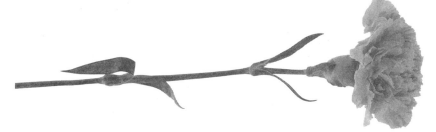

Cedarwood

Description	Originally, cedarwood oil was derived from the Lebanon cedar. However, over time and continued usage, there are not enough of these trees remaining to satisfy the demand. Presently, products are developed in Morocco from the Atlas cedar and in North America from the red cedar.
Planetary Influence	Jupiter
Secondary Planet	Uranus
Elemental Association	Air
Secondary Element	Earth
Zodiac Influence	Aries, Sagittarius
Mental/Emotional Effects	Clears confusion, calming
Healing Properties	Cleansing, health maintenance
Magickal Properties	Spirituality, purification, grounding

Cinnamon (!)

Description

For ages, the scent of this Asian tree bark has graced the culinary shelf as well as the magickal altar. It has been favored as an incense ingredient for centuries and was a highly valued commodity along the early trade routes. With such a rich history, it is unfortunate that many modern-day aromatherapists and magicians have let it slip from their list of ingredients. However, this is not without good reason. Cinnamon oil is perhaps one of the most irritating of all the essentials. Some of the more sensitive of us may find the burning sensation caused by the slightest skin contact nearly unbearable. So, although it is included in this presentation, it is imperative that its properties as an irritant are emphasized. ***Avoid direct skin contact!*** Also be aware that, should the skin come into contact with cinnamon oil, wash with cold water. Hot water will open the pores and compound the irritation.

Planetary Influence   Sun

Secondary Planet   Mars

Elemental Association   Fire

Secondary Element   Earth

Zodiac Influence   Leo

Mental/Emotional Effects   Dispels fear, awakens will and courage, removes apathy

Healing Properties   General tonic, aphrodisiac

Magickal Properties   Energy, aphrodisiac (especially for males), courage, self-confidence, strength. As a trace element in blends tends to make the overall effect stronger. Used in some cultures to attract good fortune.

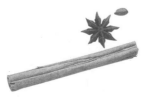

Civet

Description	Natural civet is derived from the musky secretion of an African cat. Because of cost and the necessity of destroying these animals in order to gain the essential, true civet is not readily available. There are some excellent synthetics, however, that capture the essence of the original. Here it might be noted that, in the application of synthetic oils, it is absolutely crucial to know the quality of your commercial supplier. While many oil providers do not even carry this particular scent, my contacts have uncovered two that do. One version might be a good base oil. Although it captures the spirit of the essence, it is very mild. The other is a powerfully scented blend. Where it might take an entire dram, or ⅛ ounce, of the first variation, the second would be overstated if more than 3 drops are used in an oil formula.
Planetary Influence	Venus
Secondary Planet	Mars Note: Although Mars is listed as a secondary planet, it should be understood that this is done because of its association with passion. Civet is a very female scent. While it may affect the male intensely, it is of and by the feminine nature.
Elemental Association	Earth
Secondary Element	Water
Zodiac Influence	Taurus
Mental/Emotional Effects	Awakens self-confidence (particularly in women), arouses sexuality
Healing Properties	To remedy frigidity and female sexual disorders
Magickal Properties	Attracts men (this is a female sex scent); used in combination with other love oils, it is said to make women irresistible to men

Clove (!)

Description

Another common resident of the kitchen spice rack, clove is derived from the dried flower bud of an Asian tree. It is another skin-irritating oil. Although the sensation is not as intense as that of cinnamon, the aromatherapist should be well aware that it could have ill effects if physical contact takes place.

Planetary Influence   Jupiter

Secondary Planet   Sun

Elemental Association   Fire

Secondary Element   Earth

Zodiac Influence   Cancer

Mental/Emotional Effects   Arouses courage, awakens memory, promotes clear focus

Healing Properties   Mild stimulant, used primarily in combination with other therapeutic blends to boost their effect

Magickal Properties   Courage, clarity, energy, passionate love

Cyclamen

Description

Cyclamen oil derives from the flowers of the same name. These red, white, or pink blossoms, when pressed into an essential oil, do not enjoy the popularity of many other essentials but the end product has a definite place on the shelf of the experienced magickal aromatherapist. Of the family primrose, cyclamen was once widely used as a love scent but is now more appreciated for its therapeutic virtues. It still survives in some of the old traditional magickal formulas, however, as an oil of love.

Planetary Influence	Venus
Secondary Planet	Mercury
Elemental Association	Earth
Secondary Element	Air
Zodiac Influence	Cancer
Mental/Emotional Effects	Much as this scent has an age-old reputation as a blood purifier, it tends to have a clearing effect on the mental and emotional facilities as well. It was long employed as a love oil, yet it works in a way that is unlike many of the other traditional love oils. Rather than awaken feelings of passion or arouse the soft sensitivities of appreciation of beauty, it tends to clear the mind and heart of any obstacles that may stand in the way of Cupid's endeavors. It may well stir the hot blood of passion but it does so by cleansing and not by arousal.
Healing Properties	Used for treatment of nervous disorders as well as to expel excess fluid from the system. May be used to dry congestion or relieve bloating. It is a blood purifier and also has value for the relief of insomnia, migraine headaches, coughs, and bronchitis.
Magickal Properties	Traditionally used to clear the way for love and passion, cyclamen also has another lesser-known magickal application. It is said that a single drop of cyclamen will draw the truth from anyone living in falsehood, betraying the deceptions of any liar.

Cypress

Description	The cypress tree from which this essential oil is extracted originated as an oriental plant. Over the years, however, this tree has been cultivated in many lands.
Planetary Influence	Saturn
Secondary Planet	Venus
Elemental Association	Earth
Secondary Element	Water
Zodiac Influence	Libra, Capricorn
Mental/Emotional Effects	Eases feelings of loss, instills comfort, softens impatience, eases confusion
Healing Properties	Antiseptic, antispasmodic, astringent, diuretic, sedative, vasoconstrictor
Magickal Properties	Comfort, solace

Elderberry

Description	Oil is pressed from the fruit of the elder tree. While there are several plants in the elder family, it is necessary to be aware that there are some important differences between them. This is especially true if one chooses to prepare their own essentials from the raw plant. While the American black elder yields fruit that is accommodating enough to be used in pies and preserves, the berries of the European black elder have laxative properties. The seeds contained within the fruit of the red elder are poisonous.
Planetary Influence	Venus
Secondary Planet	Saturn
Elemental Association	Water
Secondary Element	Moon

Zodiac Influence	Libra
Mental/Emotional Effects	Arouses emotions, antidepressant, boosts self-confidence
Healing Properties	General well-being, stimulant, blood purifier
Magickal Properties	Joy, happiness

Eucalyptus

Description	This is a scent familiar to anyone who has ever taken a cough drop to allay the symptoms of a cold. It is the famed staple of the koala bear. Like its well-loved devotee, the eucalyptus is native to Australia. It is of the evergreen family and is at home in Australia and Tasmania. Another variation, known as blue gum, thrives in the American soils of Florida and California.
Planetary Influence	Mercury
Secondary Planet	Saturn
Elemental Association	Air
Secondary Element	Earth
Zodiac Influence	Gemini, Aquarius
Mental/Emotional Effects	Promotes openness, trust, and clear thought
Healing Properties	Eases breathing, expectorant, antiseptic
Magickal Properties	Purification, communication, spirit contact

Frankincense

Description	Resins collected from the bark of the tree called boswellia carteri are used to produce this ancient scent. The resin, as it is collected, is in hard, pebble-like droplets. To produce the oil, these bits of resin are steamed, thereby producing the essential product.
Planetary Influence	Sun
Secondary Planet	Pluto
Elemental Association	Fire
Secondary Element	Air
Zodiac Influence	Leo, Aries
Mental/Emotional Effects	Relieves confusion and guilt, eases paranoia, promotes awareness
Healing Properties	More valuable for ailments of the mind than the body, but may enhance the effect of remedies for treatment of chronic complaints
Magickal Properties	Spirituality, success

Galangal

Description	Originating in China, galangal is a relative of the ginger root and very similar to it in its scent, appearance, and properties.
Planetary Influence	Sun
Secondary Planet	Mars
Elemental Association	Fire
Secondary Element	Earth
Zodiac Influence	Aries, Scorpio
Mental/Emotional Effects	Sparks determination and willpower, reduces fear
Healing Properties	Helps to promote quick healing, tonic, stimulant, eases symptoms of colds and congestion, promotes circulation
Magickal Properties	Courage, strength, energy, also used to win or avoid legal entanglements

Gardenia

Description	From Grandma's perfume to Mother's garden, the scent of gardenias is common to many of us. It is a common flower, plentiful, and a longtime favorite of perfumers everywhere.
Planetary Influence	Venus
Secondary Planet	Moon
Elemental Association	Water
Secondary Element	Air
Zodiac Influence	Libra
Mental/Emotional Effects	Calming, self-confidence, trust
Healing Properties	General well-being and comfort, more virtuous in the convalescing phase than the actual healing process
Magickal Properties	Love, peace, spirituality

Heliotrope

Description   While heliotrope in its own right exudes a marvelous blend of scents, a true essential is not easily obtainable. The fragrance of heliotrope seems somewhat woody, somewhat fruity, and with a hint of vanilla. Unfortunately, it does not lend itself to easy distillation. There are, however, some synthetic oils available that are very true to the spirit of the natural fragrance of the plant.

Planetary Influence	Sun
Secondary Planet	Venus
Elemental Association	Fire
Secondary Element	Earth
Zodiac Influence	Leo, Gemini
Mental/Emotional Effects	Self-confidence
Healing Properties	General well-being, health maintenance
Magickal Properties	Attraction of money, general welfare, gain power

Honeysuckle

Description   Visions of childhood years—of running along the hedges abundantly starred with the sweet white and yellow flowers—awaken with the scent of honeysuckle. The taste of the tiny blossoms' sweet nectar is not unlike the sweetness of the fragrance they carry.

Planetary Influence	Jupiter
Secondary Planet	Neptune

Elemental Association	Earth
Secondary Element	Water
Zodiac Influence	Cancer
Mental/Emotional Effects	Arouses empathy, promotes self-acceptance
Healing Properties	Aids digestion, speeds metabolism, may be utilized for weight loss
Magickal Properties	Strength, control, self-confidence, attraction

Hyacinth

Description	According to Greek myth, Hyacinthus was a youth dearly loved but accidentally killed by the god Apollo. To preserve his memory, Apollo caused the flower we now know as the hyacinth to sprout from the blood of the beloved youth. It is a flower favored for its fragrance in many gardens and survives as a lasting tribute to the ill-fated youth of the ancient myth.
Planetary Influence	Venus
Secondary Planet	Jupiter
Elemental Association	Water
Secondary Element	Earth
Zodiac Influence	Taurus, Pisces
Mental/Emotional Effects	Eases tension, guilt, and self-pity
Healing Properties	Sedative, anti-nervine, aids in cases of insomnia
Magickal Properties	Love

Jasmine

Description	The scent of jasmine is a meeting of east and west. Originally considered a blossom of the Orient, the fragrance has found a home in the American South, favored by the belles of New Orleans. Its odor is a fascinating mixture of scented tones, sweet and mysterious as well as musky in nature.
Planetary Influence	Jupiter
Secondary Planet	Moon
Elemental Association	Water
Secondary Element	Earth
Zodiac Influence	Taurus, Cancer
Mental/Emotional Effects	Overcome apathy, reduce fear, helps to relieve oversensitivity
Healing Properties	Antidepressant, aphrodisiac, insomnia
Magickal Properties	Promotes dreams and visions, general good fortune, including fulfillment of financial and romantic needs

Juniper

Description	Most often seen in essential oil form, this extract from the fruit of the juniper shrub is a cousin of the evergreen clan found growing throughout North America, Europe, and Asia. Juniper berries enjoy a wide usage and have earned a place through history in the hands of the culinary technician as well as the herbologist and the aromatherapist.
Planetary Influence	Sun
Secondary Planet	Jupiter
Elemental Association	Fire

Secondary Element	Water
Zodiac Influence	Leo, Sagittarius
Mental/Emotional Effects	Overcome obsession, relieve apathy, reduce fear
Healing Properties	Metabolic stimulant, promote weight loss, aid digestive disorders
Magickal Properties	Strength, justice

Lavender

Description	Another familiar friend, lavender originates from the Mediterranean lands but has been cultivated widely for its fragrant flowers. While it is a common addition to the repertoire of the magickal aromatherapist, it has also been an enduring favorite of cosmetic perfumery.
Planetary Influence	Mercury
Secondary Planet	Venus
Elemental Association	Air
Secondary Element	Water
Zodiac Influence	Gemini, Virgo
Mental/Emotional Effects	Dispels anxiety, removes suspicion, reduces sadness
Healing Properties	Calming, antiseptic, relieves insomnia, treatment of headaches, general health
Magickal Properties	Love, health, calm, brings peace and comfort to the home

Lemon (!)

Description

An almost universal appeal has been generated for this common scent. Its clean, fresh fragrance lends itself to teas and cleaning products as well as air fresheners and room deodorizers. The essential oil is normally procured from the peel of the fruit. It is interesting that, as aromatic as the fruit is, it takes an incredible amount of raw product to manufacture a small amount of essential oil. For this reason, much of the available lemon oil is actually made up of only a small portion of natural essential added to a synthetic base oil.

Planetary Influence	Moon
Secondary Planet	Sun
Elemental Association	Water
Secondary Element	Fire
Zodiac Influence	Cancer
Mental/Emotional Effects	Energizing, calming
Healing Properties	Stimulant, tonic, blood purifier, stomachic
Magickal Properties	Cleansing, general use for good luck and power

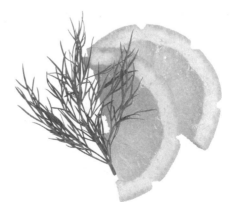

Lemon Verbena (!)

Description	Manufactured from the plant of the same name, this essential has a scent of fresh lemon mixed with herbs. In addition to its magickal and therapeutic applications, lemon verbena oil is popular in shampoos and other cosmetic body preparations.
Planetary Influence	Mercury
Secondary Planet	Venus
Elemental Association	Air
Secondary Element	Water
Zodiac Influence	Gemini, Virgo
Mental/Emotional Effects	Eases tensions, instills trust
Healing Properties	Calming, sedative
Magickal Properties	Love, trust, may be used to overcome crossed conditions

Lilac

Description	Another common scent in many gardens, lilac has been utilized in every type of commercial product from perfume to shampoo to chewing gum. In the 1960s or 1970s there was even a candy produced that used the petals of this fragrant blossom.
Planetary Influence	Venus
Secondary Planet	Uranus
Elemental Association	Earth
Secondary Element	Water
Zodiac Influence	Pisces
Mental/Emotional Effects	Comfort, security, ease
Healing Properties	Sedative, lessens anxiety
Magickal Properties	Love, ease, attracts friendly spirits for aid

Lily of the Valley

Description	Lily of the valley is native to Eurasian soil but has made its way to the gardens and countrysides throughout North America. Its soft scent makes it a favorite base oil in the perfumery as it tends to enhance rather than overpower other fragrances.
Planetary Influence	Mercury
Secondary Planet	Moon
Elemental Association	Air
Secondary Element	Water
Zodiac Influence	Gemini, Pisces
Mental/Emotional Effects	Awakens memory, instills feeling of acceptance, reduces anxiety
Healing Properties	Commonly used as a base in a variety of blends, may add a soothing quality to other treatments, thereby reducing resistance to their effects.
Magickal Properties	Peace, harmony, love

Lime

Description	A cousin to the lemon, this green fruit yields oil in much the same way as its citrus kin—from the pressed rind. It is also complementary to its relative fruit in use, and the essentials of lemon and lime blend quite well with each other.
Planetary Influence	Sun
Secondary Planet	Venus
Elemental Association	Fire
Secondary Element	Water
Zodiac Influence	Gemini, Leo

Mental/Emotional Effects	Tension reducer, tolerance enhancer
Healing Properties	Stimulant, tonic, stomachic
Magickal Properties	Cleanser, protection through spiritual favor, causes a lover to be faithful

Lotus

Description	The jeweled flower of the east has been preserved as a sacred religious symbol in Egyptian and Hindu art and literature. It is, in fact, a member of the family of water lilies. Its scent as well as its blossom have long been revered in the sacred temples of the Asian peoples.
Planetary Influence	Uranus
Secondary Planet	Moon
Elemental Association	Water
Secondary Element	(none applicable)
Zodiac Influence	Aquarius, Cancer
Mental/Emotional Effects	Self-confidence, self-acceptance
Healing Properties	May have some value in easing the transition of female hormonal change in menopause, but is chiefly a spiritual/ magickal scent
Magickal Properties	Spirituality, meditation, universal love, attracts good fortune, increases magickal power, instills longevity

Magnolia

Description Native to the Atlantic and Gulf coast states, the magnolia has taken a place in American history. The scent of this flower is highly favored throughout the South but especially in New Orleans, where it was a treasured fragrance of the women who worked in the Louisiana brothels throughout the first century of American history.

Planetary Influence Venus

Secondary Planet Uranus

Elemental Association Water

Secondary Element Earth

Zodiac Influence Taurus, Libra

Mental/Emotional Effects Arouses sexuality, reduces antisocial tendencies

Healing Properties Impotence, frigidity, general sexual disorders

Magickal Properties Love, attraction, sexual arousal, an aid to insight and understanding in meditation

Mimosa

Description	The vision of a mimosa, with its soft branches and delicate blooms, presents a dreamy picture much attuned with the magickal uses of its essential fragrance. Like the specter of its appearance, the scent of the mimosa carries us somewhere between the worlds of dream and reality to the lands rich with imagination, where poets and prophets dwell.
Planetary Influence	Saturn
Secondary Planet	Moon
Elemental Association	Air
Secondary Element	Earth
Zodiac Influence	Capricorn, Cancer
Mental/Emotional Effects	Spurs on the imagination, awakens artistic thought
Healing Properties	Clears confusion, aids in sleep disorders
Magickal Properties	Dreams, visions, hexing an enemy, ensures repayment of loans and other monies due

Muguet

Description

This is a little-known variation of lily of the valley. On last researching its origin several years ago, it became apparent that this scent has become obscure enough to have escaped from the minds of many actively working perfumers and aromatherapists. The raw flower from which the essential oil would be derived apparently grows only in a small area in France. Because of its rarity, it is seldom seen in a true essential. If it were commercially produced, it may well be a key ingredient in the famed French perfumes that sell for thousands of dollars per ounce. In fact, one perfumer estimated the cost of producing a true muguet essential at approximately $2,000 for four ounces—and that's wholesale price! As far as the synthetics are concerned, after contacting over a dozen different commercial suppliers, I only found three who claimed to produce a synthetic muguet oil. One of those actually used the names *muguet* and *lily of the valley* interchangeably, and did not offer two distinctly separate scents. Another had an actual muguet synthetic that had a very weak, diluted scent. The third seemed to understand the uniqueness of this obscure fragrance and produced a synthetic true to the spirit of the actual essential. This is difficult to find but it is priceless to those who understand and can utilize its virtue.

Planetary Influence   Venus

Secondary Planet   Mercury

Elemental Association   Air

Secondary Element   Water

Zodiac Influence   Libra

Mental/Emotional Effects   Openness, acceptance, sexual arousal

Healing Properties	May be utilized to combat sexual disorders, particularly if they are emotionally or hormonally generated
Magickal Properties	Attraction, sex

Musk

Description	Originally produced from the musk glands of animals, musk is one of the earliest fragrance aphrodisiacs. Today, with a greater awareness of preserving nature's balance and an increased kindness to the creatures who inhabit the earth, most available musk oil is synthetic. There are many variations of musk oil on the market. In fact, there is one manufacturer that lists seven different types of musk in its catalog. Most people who utilize the oil settle on one of the more adaptable versions, like sweet musk, and use it in all blends for which it is appropriate. Within my own complement of oils there are two different types of musk oil: sweet musk and earthy musk. (However, I have also come across oils presented as Egyptian musk, black musk, and African musk.) This is largely a matter of personal preference and a desire to be able to fine-tune the resulting blend rather than for absolute necessity.
Planetary Influence	Sun
Secondary Planet	Venus
Elemental Association	Earth
Secondary Element	Fire
Zodiac Influence	Leo, Sagittarius
Mental/Emotional Effects	Awakens instinct
Healing Properties	Spurs on the body's own capacity for self-healing
Magickal Properties	Passion, sex, lust; used by both sexes to attract a mate

Myrrh (!)

Description   Myrrh is one of the oldest fragrances employed in therapeutic and ritual aromatherapy pursuits. Its home is in ancient Babylonia and the biblical lands. It was no stranger to the temples of the great Egyptian culture, and was offered equally reverently to the gods who took residence on Mount Olympus. The oil is produced from the yellow-orange gum of the myrrh bush, and has been an especially favored scent for incense in ancient times. Although it is not the sweetest of fragrances (it has a musty, smoky sort of aroma), its sacred nature and ready availability in the cradle lands of religion have made it a key fragrance for perfume as well as religious observance in civilizations past.

Planetary Influence   Sun

Secondary Planet   Jupiter

Elemental Association   Fire

Secondary Element   Earth

Zodiac Influence   Scorpio, Sagittarius

Mental/Emotional Effects   Awakens spiritual zeal

Healing Properties   Menstruation, ear infections, general health

Magickal Properties   Spirituality, health, blessing; may be used for invocation of spirits, for protection, and sometimes for love

Oakmoss (!)

Description   Oakmoss grows on the trunks of oak trees. The essential product is rich with the aromas of nature, a delicate balance of sweetness and musty woods. It has hints of both soil and sea in its aroma and,

though considered a basically masculine
scent, has a soft undertone to its fragrance.

Planetary Influence	Jupiter
Secondary Planet	Saturn
Elemental Association	Earth
Secondary Element	Water
Zodiac Influence	Taurus
Mental/Emotional Effects	Security, confidence, stability
Healing Properties	Reduces hysteria, fear, anxiety, hyperactivity
Magickal Properties	Grounding, balancing, banishing

Orange (!)

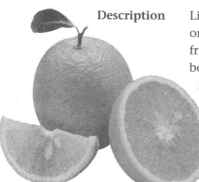

Description   Like some of the other fruity scents, the
orange essential can be derived from the
fruit, the blossom, or a combination of
both. A pure blossom essential is often
recognized by the name neroli. More
often the fragrant oil known as orange
is produced from the aromatic skin of
the fruit. Like its citrus family rela-
tives, the lemon and the lime, orange
oil is employed in a great
variety of ways, from the kitchen to the
cosmetic to the therapeutic and magickal.

Planetary Influence	Sun
Secondary Planet	Venus
Elemental Association	Fire
Secondary Element	Earth
Zodiac Influence	Leo
Mental/Emotional Effects	Arouses happiness
Healing Properties	Colds, inflammations, depression, tonic
Magickal Properties	Instills joy, happiness, energy; also used to create a harmonious, positive atmosphere

Patchouli

Description

Patchouli is native to India but is now cultivated throughout the world. It is a very potent aromatic as it is musty-sweet in small quantities yet overpowering in high volume. In the United States, the fragrance gained notable popularity as an incense and essential oil in the 1960s and 1970s. However, it first made its mark in the fashion world. In the 1800s, the scent of patchouli was used to scent woven shawls imported into the United Kingdom from India. In marketing these garments it was discovered that, while the scented garments experienced a great deal of popularity, the same product offered for sale without the scent of patchouli remained on the shelf unsold. A fascinating aspect of this bit of history is that one of the magickal applications of this essential oil is to draw money. It may give us cause to ponder whether the scent of patchouli is a faculty of marketing or magick.

Planetary Influence Saturn

Secondary Planet Mars

Elemental Association Earth

Secondary Element Fire

Zodiac Influence Taurus, Capricorn

Mental/Emotional Effects Helps to clear thought facilities, sharpen wit, relieve anxiety and depression

Healing Properties Antidepressant, antiseptic, sedative, tonic; may also be useful in the clearing and healing of skin disorders

Magickal Properties Arouses passion, attracts money

Peppermint (!)

Description

Peppermint is another plant that has the honor of mythological creation in ancient Greece. According to the legend, there was once a nymph called Mentha who was beloved of Pluto. Persephone, the mate of the underworld god, pursued the nymph in a fit of jealousy. On finding her, the goddess trampled the nymph into the ground. Through the magick of Pluto, Mentha rose again as the wonderfully fragrant plant we now know as mint. Because of its almost universal usage, peppermint oil is a staple for many who practice the arts of aromatherapy. It has its place in cooking, health, magick, and cosmetics, and is not limited to the world of arcane arts and sciences, as evidenced in its use in toothpaste, mouthwashes, teas, candies, deodorizers, and cold remedies, to name but a few.

Planetary Influence   Mercury

Secondary Planet   Venus

Elemental Association   Air

Secondary Element   Earth

Zodiac Influence   Gemini

Mental/Emotional Effects   Clears confusion, instills clarity of mind and heart, refreshes

Healing Properties   May be used in the treatment of breathing ailments such as asthma, bronchitis, colds, coughs, influenza, and sinusitis. Also useful for mental fatigue and headaches, stomach disorders, and hysteria.

Magickal Properties   May be used as a hex oil or to attract certain voodoo gods

Pine

Description	Commonly known as a key ingredient in cleaners and disinfectants, its therapeutic value parallels its household use. Easily recognized as the fragrance of "clean," it can also be used to cleanse the body and mind.
Planetary Influence	Mars
Secondary Planet	Jupiter
Elemental Association	Earth
Secondary Element	Air
Zodiac Influence	Aries, Scorpio
Mental/Emotional Effects	Raises determination, survival instinct, and the will to live; clears negativity
Healing Properties	Clears breathing, antiseptic
Magickal Properties	Increases will, determination; may be used to summon divine aid in ritual work

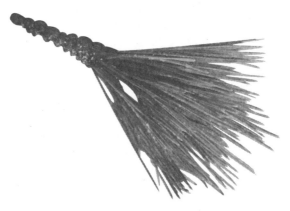

Rose

Description	When we think of roses, the picture that first comes to mind is the blood-red flower, though there are many colored variations. This is fitting, for there are many tales of the rose that relate it to blood. In varying mythologies, it is said to have risen from the blood of Venus or from the blood of Adonis. This is a fragrance that has long been appreciated for its pleasing aroma as well as its therapeutic value. In many forms, the virtue of the rose is still widely used today. In addition to the essential oil, there is rose water and tincture of rose as well as the employment of the raw petals of the blossom. While a common fragrance, its virtues have transcended time and culture.
Planetary Influence	Venus
Secondary Planet	Moon
Elemental Association	Earth
Secondary Element	Air
Zodiac Influence	Libra, Cancer
Mental/Emotional Effects	Instills harmony, eases jealousy
Healing Properties	Calming
Magickal Properties	A love oil; also addresses spirituality

Rosemary (!)

Description	One of the more common cooking spices, rosemary has also been long employed as a medicinal remedy. The therapeutic benefits of rosemary were heralded by many of the seventeenth and eighteenth century English herbalists, and the essential oil has been in common use for more than a hundred years. In modern times, there are many aromatherapists who view rosemary as a sort of heal-all remedy, good for many of the ailments that plague humankind and as a promoter of general health and well-being.
Planetary Influence	Sun
Secondary Planet	Mercury
Elemental Association	Fire
Secondary Element	Air
Zodiac Influence	Leo, Aries
Mental/Emotional Effects	Arouses memory
Healing Properties	Stimulant, liver and gall bladder treatment, aids in breathing, headache, colitis, diarrhea, treatment of burns—somewhat of a miracle remedy (some say it even cures baldness!)
Magickal Properties	Promotes longevity, general well-being, and health

Sandalwood

Description	Sandalwood is an age-old source for fragrant usage, both for religious and for therapeutic purpose. Ancient writings dating as far back as the fifth century B.C. substantiate its common usage in the land we now recognize as India. And while it is still a very popular Asian aromatic, sandalwood has become commonplace worldwide. Unlike many of the other woody scents, sandalwood oil is produced not from the bark of the host tree but from the inner wood. Although the aroma of the essential oil is decidedly woody, it has an almost bitter, musky quality to it. This is significant to note as the scent of sandalwood is suggestive of the male sex hormone androsterone. Not surprisingly, one of the magickal uses of the essential oil is to arouse passion.
Planetary Influence	Jupiter
Secondary Planet	Neptune
Elemental Association	Earth
Secondary Element	Water
Zodiac Influence	Cancer, Pisces
Mental/Emotional Effects	Eases anxiety and depression, loosens imagination, frees inhibitions
Healing Properties	Male hormones, genital and urinary tract complaints
Magickal Properties	Healing, spirituality, arouses sexual feelings

Spikenard

Description

Not one of the more common oils, spikenard nevertheless has had a long history of usage. There is a bible story that relates the tale of a devoted woman who anointed the feet of Christ with precious oil believed to be spikenard. Even at that time, as much as 2,000 years ago, this aromatic essential was dear to obtain. In today's money, it would have cost $300–$400 for a small container of the scent. Even today, spikenard oil is not one of the more common oils, and may be more obtainable in a synthetic form than as a natural essential. Many practitioners have simply eliminated spikenard from their selection of essentials. However, those who do continue to use this ancient treasure, though they may use it sparingly, value its place among their essentials very highly.

Planetary Influence	Saturn
Secondary Planet	Neptune
Elemental Association	Water
Secondary Element	Earth
Zodiac Influence	Capricorn, Pisces
Mental/Emotional Effects	Brings strength and comfort
Healing Properties	Treats migraine headaches, defeats stress, increases confidence
Magickal Properties	Brings strength, confidence, and promotes self-esteem

Strawberry

Description

Although the fruit of the strawberry is not uncommon, many of the available essential oils are synthetic. Although the purists may find some degree of impatience with the wide usage of artificial scent, this particular essential remains an extremely popular fragrance and stubbornly endures above the continued objections of the naturalist advocates. One of the factors in its continued polarity may be its association with traits that seem to be reincarnated under different names by successive generations. Strawberry has been associated with self-love but also with that which has been touted as universal love, brotherly love, free love, or unconditional love. To many, this essential, genuine or synthetic, speaks of the grand ideal of humankind. As long as men and women dream of a perfect world—a paradise on earth—the fragrance of the strawberry may continue to herald their idealistic visions.

Planetary Influence	Venus
Secondary Planet	Mercury
Elemental Association	Air
Secondary Element	Earth
Zodiac Influence	Libra
Mental/Emotional Effects	Brings joy and love of life
Healing Properties	Alleviates depression and guilt
Magickal Properties	For universal and self-love

Vanilla

Description
Common to the city dweller as well as the farm worker, vanilla spurs on many pleasantries of childhood memory. Whether it is a fragrance reminiscent of Grandma's baking or the scent of ice cream being freshly cranked, almost everyone will recall pleasant times filled with the fragrance of vanilla. Some may remember it as the aroma of snow cream, the poor folks' ice cream concocted from vanilla, a few common kitchen staples, and some freshly fallen snow. Most commonly vanilla is used in extract form for culinary pursuits, but it is also available in essential oil form. These days it has adopted a varied complement of uses, from the cosmetic preparations including shampoos, skin creams, and massage oils to the magickal, therapeutic, and flavor applications.

Planetary Influence Venus

Secondary Planet Jupiter

Elemental Association Water

Secondary Element Earth

Zodiac Influence Libra, Pisces

Mental/Emotional Effects Builds self-confidence

Healing Properties Relieves melancholy, insecurity

Magickal Properties Builds self-confidence, arouses sexual desires, brings good luck

Violet

Description	Both the flower and the leaf may be used to produce violet oil. This is another fragrance that is readily available in artificial form, as the natural product is cost prohibitive. While it is true that the leaf essential is less expensive to produce than the flower oil, neither one is cheaply manufactured. As its application affects the mental status more than the physical, violet oil is more commonly used for magickal rather than therapeutic purpose, though it is not without value in treating some conditions of the mind.
Planetary Influence	Venus
Secondary Planet	Mercury
Elemental Association	Air
Secondary Element	Earth
Zodiac Influence	Gemini, Libra
Mental/Emotional Effects	Helps overcome shyness, brings a sense of reality
Healing Properties	A calming, opening effect; may be used to aid extreme introverts
Magickal Properties	Brings peaceful conditions, opens up the psychic facilities, increases passion

Vetivert

Description	Vetivert offers a grassy, woody scent that is very clean and refreshing, like the scent of newly mown hay. It is produced from the rootstock of certain grasses and has significant application in both magickal and healing venues.
Planetary Influence	Jupiter
Secondary Planet	Uranus
Elemental Association	Earth
Secondary Element	Water
Zodiac Influence	Taurus, Scorpio
Mental/Emotional Effects	Lifts fear, strengthens against temptation
Healing Properties	Reduces anxiety, helps to relieve obsessions, mild sedative effect
Magickal Properties	Protection against enemies, magickal or otherwise

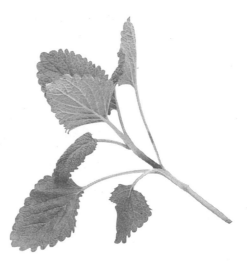

Wintergreen (!)

Description

A common scent in candies, wintergreen has developed a strong following as an externally applied treatment as well as an inhalant for aromatherapy treatment. Magickally, its uses are limited and restricted to certain cultural boundaries. The oil is one of the few that are strictly American in origin. However, therapeutically, it is gaining in popularity and use. One caution in regard to this refreshing fragrance: wintergreen should *never* be taken internally. Although this book does not promote the use of any of the listed substances through ingestion, wintergreen is poisonous enough that it is worth a special mention.

Planetary Influence Moon

Secondary Planet Mercury

Elemental Association Earth

Secondary Element Air

Zodiac Influence Cancer

Mental/Emotional Effects Has a refreshing, revitalizing, energizing effect

Healing Properties May be used to relieve muscle pain and as a catalyst for general mental and physical wellness

Magickal Properties Wisdom, general success

Ylang Ylang

Description

Ylang ylang is one of the more exotic scents. It is the fragrance of the idealist, the dreamer, the poet, and the spiritual adventurer. Even its name speaks of exotic beauty, meaning "flower of flowers." The pleasant fragrance extracted from the flowers of the ylang ylang tree lends itself to an entire array of emotional arousal. Its unique exotic fragrance makes it a favorite scent as a meditation aid for spiritual pursuit as well as a lavish ingredient connected with the pursuit of luxury in an aromatic bath. It lends itself equally well to the pleasured pursuit of godly glory and the glorious pursuit of godly pleasures. It cultivates the exotically spiritual and, as an aphrodisiac, serves the spirit of the exotic.

Planetary Influence	Venus
Secondary Planet	Mars
Elemental Association	Water
Secondary Element	Fire
Zodiac Influence	Taurus, Pisces
Mental/Emotional Effects	Calming, instills feelings of peace
Healing Properties	Hypotensor, antidepressant
Magickal Properties	Removes or reduces feelings of anger, also an ancient oil of sexual arousal

CHAPTER 6

Tools of the Trade

In most practices, all that will be needed in order
to conduct the business of oil blending will be a
selection of eyedroppers, some alcohol, vials or
other containers to house the finished creation,
and a workbook in which
to record the insights
of experimental
work, the development
of various formulae,
and any information
that may be pertinent
to research and ongoing

aromatherapy practice. While it is possible to specifically design the tools of the trade to certain criteria that may be peculiar to one way or working or another, the basic working tools listed here should suffice as a basic arsenal for the beginning aromatherapist, regardless of personal preferences and working habits. In the later stages of development, it is possible to custom design tools that may be more appropriate to a particular way of working. However, at the beginning of study, it is more important to develop a working array of tools that can be implemented by anyone, regardless of personal taste and preference.

Eye Droppers

The most vital of these tools is a selection of eye droppers, easily obtained from most drug stores, grocery stores, or chemistry dealers. The reason that several are kept on hand at all times is to keep the blends pure. When using one specific oil ingredient, it may be counterproductive to employ a dropper that has the residue of another ingredient still on it from a prior use. Rather than cleaning the dropper after every designed remedy is blended, it is easier to pick up another dropper.

Just as a hint, my own personal preference with eye droppers is to use the glass ones exclusively. Plastic droppers tend to be more porous, and may more readily retain the scents of oils. The glass droppers will wash out more easily, enabling the aromatherapist to maintain a purity of aromas by eliminating the residue from prior usage.

When it is convenient to do so, the eye droppers employed in the blending process may be cleaned. The easiest way to do this is to soak them in alcohol. The rubber bulb of the eye dropper should be removed before this is done. Otherwise, the bulb may swell and become ill-fitting and unusable. In most cases, the oils will dissolve in the alcohol and offer a clean dropper to use in the continued aromatherapy practice. However, there are some oils like amber, benzoin, camphor, and myrrh that are a bit thicker than others. These may adhere to the inside of the dropper regardless of the amount of time that they sit in a container of alcohol. For these stubborn, sticky oils it may be necessary to soak a Q-Tip in alcohol to eliminate the previous residue, but in most cases the alcohol itself will suffice to do the job. One of the marvelous things about using alcohol as a cleaning solution is that is has a very fast rate of evaporation, nearly eliminating drying time. However, if it becomes necessary to utilize the droppers before the alcohol has entirely evaporated, a Q-Tip can be used to eliminate the remaining few droplets of alcohol from the inside of the dropper.

Alcohol

While there are some aromatherapists who utilize alcohol to dilute a scent, it seems to weaken the overall effect of the blend. My own practice utilizes alcohol strictly for the purpose of cleansing. One of the most inexpensive and readily available types of alcohol is rubbing alcohol. This is satisfactory for the desired application. There are also perfumer's alcohols that are commercially available. However, the purchase of these solutions often requires a special license, and the cost is far greater than that of the rubbing alcohol that may be available at the local drugstore or supermarket. Either will act as a solvent for essential oils. The major differences are that perfumer's alcohol has no scent of its own and is far more costly than its drugstore counterpart.

Vials

Appropriately sized vials for the newly blended oil formulas, as well as a good selection of essentials from which to choose the ingredients, are all that is required to prepare for the practice of therapeutic and magickal fragrance blending.

In my own practice, I find that one dram bottles are an ideal size. While this is only an eighth of an ounce, it seems to be more than enough to last a significant length of time. As in the case of eye droppers, my own preference leans toward the use of non-porous materials such as glass. There are some who prefer amber-colored glass as a protection against the depleting rays of the sun. Some prefer the more porous containers such as those of clay. This alternative may be adequate if the container is used for the same blend, over and over. However, porous materials tend to hold on to the essence of the oil. This makes the clay containers awkward for any but the same blended fragrance. The container may retain some of the fragrance and influence of the previous resident oil, diluting the strength and intention of its present occupant. There are plastic containers that are also available, but I tend to omit these from practice. In intense or even moderate heat they tend to melt with the heating of the oil blends they may contain. Again, they are, in my opinion, too porous for ongoing usage.

In perusing the available containers that might be offered on the open market, there is a large selection of glass containers in varying sizes that might be adapted for use for aromatherapy blends. Some of these are sealed with cork stoppers, while the more expensive ones are topped with glass closures. Both may be utilized with equal effectiveness with the observation of just a few practices. First, on changing the oil blends that may be housed within the particular container, a thorough cleaning should be done to eliminate any prior scent that has been in evidence. This cleansing should include the glass stopper. In the event that the bottle was sealed by a cork, be prepared to replace this topper with another of like size. Cork is a porous material and may retain the previous scent that the glass container held.

Workbook

A final suggestion as to the practical side of aromatherapy practice would be to keep notes of your experiences. While, for the purposes of development and growth, a choice has been made to keep this formulary as a guideline to initiating a sound aromatherapy practice, most people who enter into this practice will want to build their own, more precise, formularies. Included in the workbook notes may be such information as why a decision was made to be more or less heavy-handed with this ingredient or that, or why altering a particular component or amount of a specific oil in a formula helped to customize the blend to a particular individual or situation, thereby maximizing its effectiveness. The results of specific formulas might also be tracked in the aromatherapist's personal notebook. Going back over these notes will help guide the aromatherapist to the most and least effective formulas and keep the practice of the art ever alive, ever new, and constantly developing into greater plateaus of successful practice.

Mental Tools

Of paramount importance to the art of blending scent, also, are the criteria that might be utilized for the inclusion or omission of specific ingredients. There are several basic approaches to aromatherapy blending to obtain the desired result. Some practitioners follow the virtues of the various essential oils in accordance with astrological correspondences. Some adhere to the elemental virtues. Others may pay close attention to traditional usage. Still others have molded their practices from a combination of the different virtue associations. All of these systems have merit. The final judge of a blend has less to do with the methods used for its creation than with its effectiveness in actual application. One may consider the systems of virtue associations to be guidelines in the art of blending. However, in the final analysis, an effective blend is one that works. No matter how sound the principles used to formulate a certain blend, its only true worth is seen in its final use.

As a reference to the creative oil artisan, a number of tables are included in the appendix of this volume. There are correspondence tables that offer associations of various essential oils in accordance with elemental and astrological virtues. There are also tables listing the more common irritant oils and carrier oils. These, especially, should be observed closely. There are many people who are sensitive to one oil or another. The responsible artisan will be on the watch for the individual's reaction to a particular oil or oil blend. However, there are certain essentials that carry a greater potential for irritation than others. These oils should be utilized with the greatest of caution. Carrier oils, on the other hand, are oils that are agreeable to most individuals and can be used as a base oil with little side effect. They, more than many other essentials, may be noted as user friendly.

CHAPTER 7

The Amounts

As far as the actual physical preparation of an aromatherapy blend is concerned, the original method learned twenty years ago is as valid and workable in my own practice as it ever was. Personal preference demands that blending be done in small quantities. Although many essential oils have a considerably lengthy shelf life, my own preference is to have each blend as fresh as possible. For this reason, no more than one dram of oil is prepared at a time.

The entire blending process may be considered parallel to the distillation process for the initial gathering of the essential oil itself. Raw material (the various criteria for choosing an essential fragrance) is gathered. It is then processed down (the selection process of what ingredients to include). And the end product is generated—the pure essential or resulting blended formula. It is like placing all the criteria into a large screen and producing a fine, pure, and effective fragrance.

As to the makeup of specific blends, or recipes for essential products, there are many foundational principles that may be employed. The purpose of this presentation is not to offer blind methods but to offer insights into ways that may be employed and to encourage individual expression of the art of aromatherapy. For this reason, and but for the inclusion of a few sample blends for illustration, there is no hard and fast method of blending, no specific amounts of ingredients that must be used in formulas. What is presented here are examples of what aromatherapy is capable of producing. To limit one's blends to those included in this volume is also to place restrictions on the scope of possibilities inherent in aromatherapy. The intention is to offer this writing as a springboard to greater and more effective creations in aromatherapy blends, to help aid in the understanding and continued development of the art of scent to its fullest capacity, and to serve as a foundation in exploring the farthest reaches of the possibilities of aromatherapy in the arena of healing and in its applications in magickal rites.

That being said, there is a general approach that has proven effective on a personal level of working with fragrances. This approach has resulted in blends that are both effective and unique. In fact, there have been some who have unsuccessfully tried to copy some of the more effective formulas but, because of the specific methods of creating a formula, were unable to do so. Because of the continued success of this particular method, it is offered here as a general guideline for consideration. It is not expected to be followed exactly at all times, but modified in accordance with the needs of the situation and the inspiration of the aromatherapy artisan.

Looking at the actual procedures for blending essential oils in aromatherapy, most commonly, formulas are written in very precise amounts. Generally those formulas that you see in print will have an exact number of drops for each ingredient included in a specific therapeutic or magickal oil blend. One of the major source books for magickal oil blending, however, contains only a listing of the component oils with few specific amounts for any of the individual oils. While this presentation serves as little more than a guideline in the production of the desired oil blends, it does have one benefit that we cannot enjoy in the manufacture of formulas delineated in precise ingredient proportions: it encourages, and perhaps demands, the use of the aromatherapist's own knowledge and creativity. Rather than a technical assistant for the knowledge and development of some other previously practiced and published aromatherapist, the individual artisan must utilize his or her own knowledge of the art to produce workable blends suited to a specific purpose.

The presentation in this volume is something in between the two aforementioned types of offering. While it is the intention to encourage individual skill and expression in the formulation of aromatherapy blends, a bit more than a list of ingredients has been included as a guide for the user of this formulary. In this way, a blend resulting from the given material in this work will emerge as a workable remedy or magickal product but will still have the creative touch of the individual artisan woven into its composition.

The looser presentation of the amounts of each ingredient will also allow for the fine-tuning of a particular blend to the specifics of the situation at hand or to the individual for whom it is intended. In this way, each blend of essential oils can have its own character and be custom-fitted for the particular situation, ailment, or condition that demands its employment.

On a practical level, the different essential oil ingredients are typed into three different categories. These are major components, minor influences, and trace elements. These will be noted throughout the formulary with the notations MA, mi, and T, respectively. This approach to blending has proven highly successful in my own working, and has the benefit of constantly testing the knowledge, skill, and creativity of the individual aromatherapist. Every resulting formula is a living, changeable tool. Each new design demands the constant awareness of the background principles of aromatherapy and the sensitivity of the fragrance artist. Each new blend encourages the continued learning and growth of the aromatherapist.

To look at the three categories more in depth, here is a hypothetical case where, for the purpose of example, we may assume our magickal undertaking is to restore love and stability in a shaky relationship. The major influences might be oils of Venus, or love oils. There may be more than one of these included, depending on the judgment and inspiration of the aromatherapist. These would be included in the formula in the greatest quantity. A secondary influence might be a stabilizing force, or oils of earth. The quantities of these ingredients would be less that those chosen as the

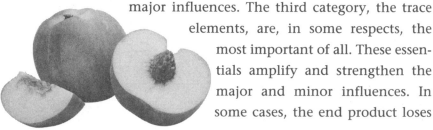

major influences. The third category, the trace elements, are, in some respects, the most important of all. These essentials amplify and strengthen the major and minor influences. In some cases, the end product loses effectiveness if the trace elements are not included. These are also the elements that make the formulas nearly impossible to copy. They serve as undertones. While only a drop or two might be included in the blend, their inclusion is often the factor that gives the end mixture its level of success.

The key to the trace elements is that because of the small amount that is used, they tend to work on a subconscious level to achieve the desired result. In this particular case, suppose we include, in trace amounts, one of the fragrances that are akin to naturally produced scents of passionate arousal. Since we are dealing with a relationship that has been ongoing, there is likely love already in evidence. We enhance that existing feeling with the love oils. We interject a note of stability to help the couple weather the difficult times. The inclusion of the arousal scents can act to rekindle the flame that may have been cooled in the stresses of day-to-day difficulties. The end result is that, while the conscious reaction to the magickal blend would be to remember the bonds of love and gain a sense of strength and stability through uncertain changes, the unconscious reaction would be a strengthening of the passions that bind the couple together. With these feelings rekindled, there may still be tough times in the days ahead but, with hearts bound as one, there is little question that the two individuals will face each trial together. From out of the depths of their passion is borne a deep commitment, one to the other.

The greatest benefit of this type of formulary is to ensure that learning and growth continue as the practice of the aromatherapist develops. In this way the quality and effectiveness will also continually increase, much to the advantage of those for whom the art is practiced. This should, ideally, be the goal of anyone who would undertake the practice of the ancient art of fragrance blending. Neither art nor science has ever reveled in stagnation but ever attains to greater levels of expertise and accomplishment.

These are the goals of magickal aromatherapy—to approach each endeavor on as many levels and as deeply as possible. With the strength of the virtues of the essentials, we work from the outside in and from the inside out. We touch both the conscious and the unconscious. We arouse the rational, the emotional, the thoughts, and the instincts.

By the nature of the fragrance art, the aromatherapist is accomplished artisan and inspired magician. By the responsibility of magickal working, the artisan is also humanitarian. This is the highest purpose of aromatherapy, whether applied magickally or therapeutically. It is not difficult to manipulate with fragrance, but to utilize aroma to build, develop, and fulfill the greatest potential of each individual is an expression of the fragrance artisan and of the art itself in the highest degree.

CHAPTER 8

How to Apply Scent

In the most basic translation, aromatherapy is the art of healing through aromatic substances. Yet, in application, the art of scent treatment has a dual action. Through instinctual response, like that of an animal that is equally aware (and equally stimulated) by the scent of an approaching enemy or a potential mate, our sense of smell is connected to a whole array of inborn response mechanisms. Our gut reaction to this smell or that is a touch of the wonder and bounty of nature's design.

In the case of the two-legged breed of animal, however, we have managed to open up an entirely new arena in the world of scent. We have, in addition to instinct, the reaction to the fragrances of experience. Ask yourself why one person may adore the scent of roses while another does not favor the smell. Perhaps one relates the scent to a first love, to a pleasant place, or to the memory of a beloved grandfather who spent endless hours tenderly caring for his precious rose garden. The other may recall the scent as it relates to a nasty encounter with the thorns of the rose bush or the sting of the insects that concealed their nesting place among the fabulous crimson blooms.

It is widely accepted that the physiological body has the ability to heal itself of any number of ailments. In fact, many medical doctors approach viral infection by relieving the symptoms of the illness and letting the virus run its course. In other words, we as doctors can do little in this case, so let's make the patient as comfortable as possible while the immune system does its work. With this precept as a foundation, it is easy to see that the mental/emotional state of the patient is inescapably tied to the physical healing process. For this reason, it is difficult to reasonably consider the physical and emotional processes as independent of one another. However, there are specific physical workings that are at work. For the purpose of greater understanding, we will set out to separate these inseparable workings.

Consider the inhaler devices that are in constant reach of those who suffer from serious problems with asthma, or nasal sprays in common usage by cold sufferers. While the medications utilize the mucous membranes as entryways for the remedy's introduction to the body, it should be remembered that these are the same membranes that serve to accept fragrance for transmittal to the brain. And what exactly is fragrance but airborne trace particles of its host?

Consider, also, some of the methods used in the application of aromatherapy treatments. It is important to see how they operate physiologically—for example, let's take a closer look at two of the methods of enacting aromatherapy remedies: massage and the aromatic bath.

Massage is direct application of an essential oil or oil blend to the body. (*Warning*: Not all oils can or should be applied directly to the skin. Check with your supplier.) This takes advantage of the virtues of massage therapy as well as aromatherapy. And while the scent may well act as a catalyst to spur on the immune system to its full strength in the combat of a particular ailment, it should be remembered that the essential oil is, by application directly to the skin, being absorbed into the body through the pores. It may be noted that many prefer to use heated oils in massage. Not only is this more comfortable for the recipient of the therapy, but heat acts to open up the pores and make them more receptive to the essential blend.

The use of the aromatic bath is similar. Baths are generally warm, again opening the pores to be more receptive to the essential oils used. Also, as in massage, there is direct physical contact with the body. Although the full potency of the essential is diluted by the volume of bath water, it is a direct physical application of the aromatherapy remedy. It is in this particular function that aromatherapy is easily related to the practice of homeopathy. In homeopathic practice, in order to strengthen a remedy, it is further diluted. So it is in aromatherapy that a diluted application of an essential fragrance can serve as a very potent remedy. And, through the physical workings of the art, the effectiveness of the therapy is multiplied in that it attacks an ailment on multiple levels.

Upon the design of a new oil blend, the next task is in deciding how to deliver the fragrance to the client. Which method is used is often dictated by the particulars of the situation to be remedied, or the comfort of the individual undergoing the therapy, or the preference of the aromatherapist. Ideally, the chosen application is a result of all of these considerations.

There are a number of ways to accomplish this. Some are exclusive to the therapeutic expressions of the art; others are more in keeping with the magickal aspects of aromatherapy. Although there are variations of the different application procedures of the aromatherapist, in general terms, the virtues of fragrance are transmitted through the mediums of inhalation, direct external contact, or some combination of both methods.

Note: Whether the intention of the fragrance artist is therapeutic or magickal, there are general guidelines that might be followed. These are clarified in the following pages, along with the appropriate general formulas for their preparation. Now that we have covered the why, it is time to get on to the how.

In addressing the direct application of aromatic oils to the body, it is important to emphasize the importance of knowing the physical properties of the essentials as well as their virtues for use in aromatherapy. Keep in mind that there are many oils that act as irritants to the skin. Some of the more common of these to safeguard against are:

> anise, bergamot, camphor, cassia, chili pepper, cinnamon, clove, citronella, lemon verbena, melissa, oakmoss, orange, peppermint, rosemary, wintergreen

While some may not be sensitive to these essentials, others will react extremely negatively to contact. At times, an extreme dilution into a low scent, user-friendly carrier oil will allay any discomfort. However, this is not a guaranteed way of circumventing the problem. It is also important to keep in mind that, in addition to the irritant properties of some essentials and blends, there are individual allergies to be considered. What might be a pleasing, beneficial remedy to one individual may initiate a severe allergic reaction in another. These cautions appear in more than one place in this volume, as the importance of responsibly considering these dangers cannot be understated.

Further to the gravity of the responsibility of the practicing aromatherapist is a word of advice. Be aware. Expect the improbable. Several years ago, there was an individual who had an allergic reaction to a very mild, normally universally pleasing scent. Of course, the first action taken was to immediately discontinue the use of the fragrance. But on closer investigation, it appears that there never was an allergic response to the essential. The allergy was to the carrier oil in which it had been diluted. Carrier oils are specifically chosen for their low fragrance and universal acceptability. However, though we can easily register what works for most, each individual comes complete with their own set of personal reactions, allergies, sensitivities, and tolerances. Each individual is, after all, an individual. Be aware!

Some of the formulae call for dilution of the essential blend in a carrier oil. For a complete listing of oils that make suitable carriers, refer to the appendix pages. For now, it is only important to emphasize the criteria by which carriers are chosen. When selecting a carrier, it should be one that does not interfere with the properties of the active essential. Generally, low-scent or no-scent oils are chosen so that the remedy will have its full effect and not be modified by the introduction of an alien aroma (i.e., that of the carrier oil). We want an oil that is fairly medium consistency. Too heavy or too light may not be conducive to a well mixed, evenly distributed blend, or may be difficult to administer. Not all aromatherapists favor the use of carrier oils. Whenever possible, some tend to use a lesser amount of the essential blend full strength, particularly in producing aromatic baths. However, the inclusion of carrier oils is made here. The newer practitioners of the art may find that using the carrier solution will make the remedy easier to produce and easier to apply.

So, to begin, we have the general formulae. These will become important as the comfort level and the degree of knowledge that an individual practitioner has develops and increases. At that point, it is likely that the gifted mind of the artisan will emerge, and there will be a desire to improve upon, experiment with, embellish, and re-invent the basic remedies listed here.

Therapeutic Applications

In aromatherapy practice, healing methods may employ fragrance in a number of ways. The ultimate purpose is to deliver the virtues of the scent to the client in a way that will most benefit his or her condition to ease or alleviate the complaint. Depending on the nature of the specific ailment, different methods of delivery may be chosen.

In therapeutic use, the chief methods of application include direct or indirect inhalation in combination with a soothing bath, as in a fragrant bath salt, direct local application, or in conjunction with massage therapy. Each of these methods has its own set of preparatory procedures to be followed before a given remedy is applied.

In the pages that follow also are the general formulas that will be employed for turning an oil remedy into the desired form for the intended type of delivery to the subject. These combinations are more specific in regard to the amounts of each ingredient listed—as they must be, for this is the preparation of the medium. The skill and creativity of the aromatherapist are employed in the creation of the remedy. These formulas will just place those carefully designed blends in usable form.

Direct Application

⌒ *Direct Application Formula*

5–7   drops pure essential oil, oil blend, or direct application oil
1–2   teaspoons carrier oil

Alternatively, oil may be mixed well into 1–2 teaspoons of unscented body cream, lanolin, or aloe vera cream instead of carrier oil. Be certain it is mixed thoroughly.

In some cases, an aromatherapy remedy can be applied directly to the affected area, particularly in the case of muscle ailments. A word of caution: do not apply the remedy to an area where the skin is broken! Many oils are not meant to be introduced directly into the bloodstream, plus, the danger of a negatively sensitive reaction to the remedy is increased. Again, it is imperative that the responsible aromatherapist know well the properties of the remedy and the sensitivities of the client. Because of the increased danger of negative reaction, dilutions are often used for direct application.

If the oil is not an irritant, and the subject displays no negative reaction to inhalation or skin contact with the specific remedy, sometimes the blend is rubbed into the skin directly beneath the nose. In this way, inhalation therapy can be accomplished without interruption of other daily activities. It is accomplished with every natural breath rather than through a treatment session. At this point, it would be appropriate to introduce one of the creative innovations that has arisen through the actual practice of aromatherapy. Many aromatherapists love to see men approach them for consultation sporting mustaches. Putting the inhalation treatment oil on the natural growth of facial hair beneath the nose not only allows the completion of inhalation therapy in a natural way but has the added benefit of keeping the oil away from direct skin contact. Although there is always a mandate to be aware of client responses, and it is always necessary to observe the proper precautions and maintain a high level of responsibility, this type of administration often allows the aromatherapist to employ some components in a blend that would be ill-advised for direct skin contact.

Other direct inhalation methods include inhaling the fragrance of the oil blend directly from the bottle or soaking cotton balls or cotton swabs with the remedy, holding them beneath the nostrils and inhaling the scent. This practice is undergone for up to twenty minutes at a time. Depending on need and the nature of the condition to be remedied, the process may be repeated several times throughout the day. In following this method of application, it should be noted whether the blended oil includes any irritant ingredients. While direct contact to the skin is inadvisable with some essential oils, consider how much more of an irritation might be experienced through inhalation. The nasal tissues can be very delicate and extremely sensitive. In some cases, especially when the ailment being treated is respiratory, it may be desirable to inhale the scent through the mouth instead of, or in addition to, the nose. The downside of this is the possibility of an unpleasant assault on the taste buds.

Indirect Inhalation

Another type of inhalation is an indirect method. Rather than administering the oil remedy directly to the subject, the person's surroundings are treated with the chosen scent. This can be accomplished in several different ways.

Indirect Inhalation Formula

Pure essential oil or oil blend

Oil Diffusers

> Pure essential oil or oil blend

The oil diffuser is an item developed specifically for use in diffusing essential scents into the air. It does this through breaking up the oil blend and delivering the scent into the air. These are far more costly than the simple light rings but do seem to be more effective. Like many such items, it is possible to spend a little or a lot, depending on the specific brand, construction, and special features of the particular piece of equipment purchased.

Vaporizers

> Pure essential oil or oil blend

A personal choice over the more costly oil diffuser is the vaporizer. This is the common medical device that many of us may recall as the source of the aroma of a medicated eucalyptus scent in childhood days at the onset of cold and flu season. Just place the blend in the compartment that is reserved for medication and let the vaporizer do the rest. There are both hot air and cool air vaporizers commercially available. While my own preference is to employ the cool mist type, either could accomplish the intended purpose.

Spray Mist

100–150   drops of essential oil (¾–1 dram)
   4–5   fluid ounces of water (distilled is preferred)
⅛–¼   dram alcohol (ONLY if needed to thin out some of the thicker essentials to produce a more usable spray mist. The exact amount may be varied depending on the aromatic strength of the essential. This is included only to help the mix, and should not result in an alcohol smell).

Dilute the essential blend into a spray mist and scent the home or office. This is done by mixing a small amount of the essential oil with water. Place the solution in a spray bottle (readily available at grocery, hardware, gardening supply, and many other stores) and use as one would use a commercial room freshener.

⁓ *Light Rings*

Pure essential oil or oil blend

The light ring is one of the most inexpensive aides that can be employed. It is a circlet, often made of brass with an absorbent, changeable insert, or sometimes constructed of a porous material such as clay. The ring is placed over a light bulb, and the essential oil placed in the ring. Heat from the light gently evaporates the oil into the air, scenting the entire room. As far as which type is better, it is largely a matter of preference. While the clay type of ring eliminates the need for changing the absorbent inserts, it does have a drawback in that a scent can become ingrained in the porous material. This will leave an undertone aroma of the previous usage when the oil is changed to a different purpose. These rings are normally very inexpensive and readily obtainable from almost anyone who deals with essential oil products.

⁓ *Potpourri*

Pure essential oil or oil blend

Caution should be used. Only a few drops will be required. Using more may smother the charcoal, if using an incense base. Also remember that oil products are flammable! In ancient times, before the availability of a wide range of essential oil products, the raw herbs were burned in order to deliver the virtues of the fragrance to a client. A more modern variation of this practice would be to use a potpourri pot. Oil may be added to a favorite blend, thereby delivering healing properties at the same time as pleasantly scenting the home.

⁓ *Incense*

Pure essential oil or oil blend

A similar application of this method would be to add a few drops of a healing oil blend to a favorite incense. While these methods will accomplish the purpose, it should be remembered that the scents of the potpourri or incense may create some effects of their own. The properties of these base scents may diminish, alter, or even reverse the virtues of the blended remedy. Therefore, it is wise to know the properties of the base scents, as well as the remedy, before introducing it as a viable medium for inhalation therapy.

Direct External Contact and Inhalation

Massage Therapy Oil

¼ dram essential oil
1½–2 tablespoons carrier oil

Often, the virtues of other healing disciplines are combined with aromatherapy. Of these, the most commonly seen is massage therapy. The virtues of fragrance, in combination with the benefits of massage therapy, may increase the effectiveness of the administered healing. For this, an appropriate massage oil must be produced. This is done by diluting the oil remedy with a carrier oil. There is a list of suitable carrier oils in the appendix.

Aromatherapy massage becomes more or less effective depending on the practitioner's strength of knowledge in the field of massage therapy. The accomplished masseuse can incorporate the virtues of both facets of the healing arts to maximize the overall effectiveness of the remedy.

Further possible variations of the aromatherapy massage include the practice of specific massage disciplines. The healing properties of aromatherapy may be combined with reflexology and shiatsu as well as the more mainstream expression of massage therapy. This will allow the particular ailment to be approached from more than one direction. With the increased benefit of combined healing arts, the remedy may be effected that much more quickly.

Some preparations may be applied directly to an affected area. A specific example is a bruise oil blend. While it should eventually prove helpful as an inhalant, if applied directly to the inflamed area, there seems to be an almost immediate response to the remedy. The discomfort, in many cases, begins to lessen upon the very first application, and the total time for complete elimination of the complaint is drastically reduced from the normal recovery time without the use of aromatherapy.

⌒ *Scented Baths*

15–20   drops ($\frac{1}{8}$ dram) essential oil or oil blend
$\frac{3}{4}$ dram carrier oil
$1\frac{1}{2}$–3   ounces Epsom salt

Be certain that this is mixed very thoroughly, as the oil may have a tendency to form into clumps in the salt. Even distribution is required. Also note that this will make several baths. It only takes $1\frac{1}{2}$ to 2 teaspoons of mixture for an entire bath.

While there are different preferred methods for preparing the aromatic baths, two of them emerge as the easiest and least complicated in the preparatory stages. One is to introduce the essential oil or oil blend into a small amount of Epsom salts, and to dissolve the salts into a tub of hot or warm water. Some take the trouble to add color and fixatives to the mixture to produce something comparable to the commercially available bath salts. Unless the intention is to market the end product, this is really unnecessary. In fact, the salts can be prepared in just minutes prior to the time of use.

If the essential oil blend contains ingredients that may act as irritants, you may be able to still utilize their virtuous properties if you increase the amount of Epsom salt and introduce a carrier oil to dilute the oil blend. However, if you are not certain that you can eliminate the negative effects of the irritants, it may be wiser to choose another method of administering the remedy altogether.

Another method of creating an aromatic bath is to introduce the essential blend directly into the bath water. Although this is a viable way to prepare a bath quickly, it is not the choice method for optimum effectiveness. Because oil and water do not truly mix, it is easier to get an even distribution of the fragrance if a moment is taken to mix the essential with the bath salts before adding it to the water.

Like heated massage oil, the warmth of the freshly drawn bath serves to open the pores of the skin. Thus, in addition to the benefits of inhalation while immersed in the scented water, the individual is actually taking in the healing properties of the essential blend through the skin. Aromatic baths are used in many of the available applications of the fragrance arts. They can be directed toward ritual, toward healing mind, body, and spirit, or as a lavish way of pampering oneself to beauty and elegance.

Magickal Applications

Magickal application also involves a limited number of traditional transmittal methods for employing the virtues of fragrant blends. Perfume oils may be prepared to be worn by the subject of the magickal aromatherapy endeavor. These may take two forms. One is designed to exert influence on the wearer of the scent. The other may be intended to influence those who may come in contact with the aromatherapy subject. Oil blends may also be used in connection with magickal rites. Such is the case when employing a scent in an incense, ritual bath, or in anointing the person or a symbol of the person with the scented blend (as in the case of sympathetic candle magick). In addition, fragrances may be produced as magickal powders, waters, or floor washes. In theory, any blend may be employed in any of these mediums. However, there are certain traditional applications that are often observed. As in all aromatherapy practice, however, the magickal aromatherapist must remain sensitive to the particulars of the situation at hand and employ skill and creativity in devising the best way to remedy the problem at hand, too.

Some of the more clever ways that have been used to deliver a magickal fragrance to its destination involve such tactics that some people may not be aware that some magickal influence has been exerted on their behalf. A few drops of oil may be added to the laundry of the subject. While it is diluted enough by the wash water to avoid oil stains and overpowering aromatic evidence, the subtle residue continues to influence the subject throughout every waking hour of every day. Another creative method of application has been to treat the bedsheets with the desired magickal blend. When the benefactor of the magickal virtue of the scent drifts off to sleep, the oil blend will work its magick through the night, delivered right into the subconscious thought of the unsuspecting subject.

The magickal use of aromatherapy, like its healing applications, has a limited number of common methods of delivery. The chosen method may depend, in part, on what type of magick is to be used. In general, there are three different types of magickal processes that may be practiced. The first is tied to the will and intention of the magician. Effect is generated by a pure extension of will. This is energy raised from within and directed to its purpose. Oil preparations used in this kind of magickal working may be for the enhancement of the magician as much as for the traditional effect that the magickal blends might exert on outside situations.

The second type of working is related to the will of the magician but is based on the magickal principle of creating an effect on a symbolic representation of the person or situation to be altered, thereby initiating an effect on the intended recipient of the change as well. This is known as sympathetic magick, and is the root workings of many well-known magickal disciplines, such as voodoo. The traditional voodoo doll is a prime example of this kind of working.

The final type of magickal undertaking involves the use of forces and energies outside of the practitioner. This may include the enlisting of the aid of fairies, demons, angels, spirits, or actual deities. In this kind of working, the oil blends employed may be made of scents sacred to one entity or another.

There are a number of different transmittal systems of the fragrant blends. There are several mediums that may be prepared for specific types of use, and certain methods for the employment of the magickal blends once they have been prepared.

Some of the more common methods of application are the wearing of the fragrance by the subject (again, be careful of irritants!) or, if the scent is to act upon someone other than the petitioner, the introduction of the blend into the surroundings of the person on whom it is intended to create an effect. Oils may also be used to anoint candles or symbolic representations if the undertaking falls under the trappings of sympathetic magick. In the case of the use of fragrance to honor or for the appeasement of outside forces or entities, a more ritual approach may be taken, such as the introduction of the scent into the ritual incense.

Some of the possible mediums that may be produced for the application of magickal oils are perfume oil, anointing oil, fragrant bath, scented waters, floor washes, spray mists, incense, and sprinkling powders. The general formulas for the production of these types of products are presented here.

Direct Application

Perfume Oil

Pure essential oil

Although there are some perfume oils produced by the addition of the essential blend into a solvent, like alcohol, the pure essentials will serve well. As always, the responsible aromatherapist will be on guard for irritant qualities in the components of the specific magickal formulas. This effect may be lessened by the use of a carrier oil for a base.

⌒ *Anointing Oil*

Pure essential oil

Be aware that anointing oil may be used for application to an inanimate symbolic representation of a person or directly on the individual. If the preparation is to come into contact with the skin, the appropriate observations and cautions should be observed.

Indirect Application

⌒ *Scented Waters*

7–8	drams pure essential oil or oil blend
3½–4	quarts water (distilled water is a personal preference)
¼–¾	cup alcohol

⌒ *Floor Washes*

1	gallon commercial floor cleaner (if a concentrate, enough to make one gallon of solution)
4–7	drams pure essential oil or oil blend

Be careful. This preparation is used to treat the living surroundings by washing the floor with it. Too much oil will leave a dangerous, slippery residue on the floor, which may result in physical mishaps for those who walk on the treated surface.

⌒ *Spray Mist*

100–150	drops of essential oil (¾–1 dram)
4	fluid ounces of water
	alcohol (ONLY if needed to thin out some of the thicker essential oils to produce a smoother product)

This mixture is applied using a normal water spray bottle.

Incense

50–100 drops pure essential oil or oil blend
1–1½ ounces powdered base (Two base incenses that seem to work
particularly well are cedar dust and ground orris root)

Sprinkling Powders

50–100 drops pure essential oil or oil blend
⅔–1½ ounces powder base

There are a variety of powders that may be used. The base should not
be as granular as the base used for incense, but not so fine as the
powders used cosmetically, like talcum powder or dusting powder,
either. Many prefer ground herbs like orris root or gum mastic. There
is at least one practitioner that swears by ground galangal root. In a
desperate situation with no
other substance readily
available, I've seen ground corn
meal used as an effective powder base.
However, many prefer to steer clear of
foodstuffs to avoid the inevitable
attraction of our creeping, crawling friends
that may view it as an opportunity to feast.

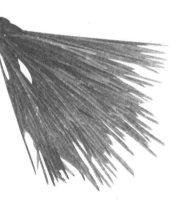

CHAPTER 9

*I*nfluences in Blending Oils

*L*ike any other discipline, whether creative,
scientific, mechanical, athletic, or within the
bounds of any other classification, aromatherapy
practice is founded on some basic guiding
principles and techniques.
The art of blending essential
oils for the optimum
results in the pursuit of
a desired effect has
certain features
unique unto itself.

The roots of the practice of aromatherapy are ancient. As such, there are many blends that have been handed down from generations that have comprised something of a traditional base of the practice. For example, the scents of frankincense and myrrh have been used in religious ceremony since the time of the ancient Egyptian culture and, very possibly, even earlier. These scents are still utilized in much the same way today. If we look at the associations of the scents in modern aromatherapy practice, it is easy to find the link of our present-day usage to the ancient practices of our ancestors.

Both of these scents are still connected in magickal practice with spirituality. If we look at their use in therapeutic aromatherapy, their applications are not unrelated to their ancient associations. Frankincense may be used to develop awareness, relieve confusion, and instill a sense of forgiveness for a condition of guilt. Religious practice is aimed at the opening of the mind of the individual to faith, the granting of comfort to the ailing soul through trust in the divine, and the acceptance and correction of past sins through spirituality and understanding. The magickal and therapeutic applications of this ancient scent are inseparable from one another.

Similarly, myrrh is also still regarded magickally as a scent of spirituality. On the therapeutic side, it is used as a general healer. As it is applied as a fragrance to restore physical health, myrrh has been used for centuries in ritual to aid in the restoration of the soul's well-being. We remain tied to the wisdom of ancient perfumers. While we may have considerably expanded the practice of aromatherapy over the years, the basic wisdom handed down by our predecessors has been the solid foundation on which we have built our modern-day blends.

Pure Essentials and Blends

Some artisans of the aromatics choose to utilize the assets of an essential oil in its fullest, purest sense. These are avid followers of single scent therapy. This approach avails the recipient of the fragrance the full virtue of the essential and allows the substance to serve its full purpose unencumbered. Without a doubt, this school of thought is not without merit.

The purist philosophy, however, is not the only approach to the use of aromatherapy. Many practicing aromatherapists choose to blend the properties of different essentials. This can serve a dual purpose. First, in the arena of healing, there are many multiple-symptom ailments that may require attention. For example, in cases where there is an apparent respiratory disorder, there may be some coughing, sneezing, and congestion. It may be appropriate to utilize an essential scent that clears breathing. But, perhaps, this ailment is accompanied by fever, headache, general weakness, or aches and pains. There may be other scents that are better suited as fever reducers, pain relievers, or tonics. This is where the process of blending essentials comes into play.

In addition, combining one scent with another could serve to modify the overall effect of the remedy. Take, for instance, the scent of eucalyptus, commonly used to clear breathing. Add a touch of lavender and the resulting blend will help to clear the confused feeling left by a stuffy head. A bit of orange oil may act as a tonic. The resulting effect of the blend would be not only to relieve the symptom of congestion but to help the suffering individual feel better, as well. Presumably, the clear, refreshed state of the client will help to speed along the ultimate recovery.

And the client's state of mind should not be underestimated. It has been said that hospitals are the worst place for recovery because they reek of sickness and so offer no inspiration but rather perpetuate illness. There is certainly no intention to downplay the healing that does go on in the sickhouses, but many would prefer to be in the comfort of familiar surroundings and positive attitudes. The quality of the attitude itself can be a marvelous catalyst to speedy recovery. Just as it is difficult to freely feel and express joy in a room filled with those wrapped in the throes of sorrow, it is difficult to find health in a place that is home to the suffering and the infirm.

This precept can be readily seen in taking a page from my own experiences in younger years. There was a man named Otto who lived near the town in which I spent much of my youth. He was a handyman by trade, earning his living through whatever household tasks one of the local families might offer, and one of the most driven and optimistic people I've met. As far as anyone knew, Otto never held a regular job. After speaking a little with him, and at great length with the adults in my life, it was revealed that Otto could not keep a regular job. His body was riddled with cancer. He was too high a risk for anyone to hire on as a permanent employee. In fact, his doctors had told him that he had only a few months left to live. As dismal as Otto's situation seemed, it really was not without hope—for the doctors had given him this diagnosis ten years earlier! Not before meeting Otto, and not since that time, have I met anyone with such an incredible will to live.

So while some will adhere strictly to the single purity of scent in aromatherapy application, some of us find greater virtue in utilizing blends. Blended essentials afford us the benefit of addressing mind and spirit as well as the physical condition, priming the natural instincts to rise to the task of self-healing. As honorable as the intention is of the aromatherapy purist, as virtuous as the art, and as noble the artisan, the possibilities that are opened by blending essentials are worthy of note. One has to wonder if the purists would be as adamant in protecting the virtues of the single scent approach to therapy if they could have known Otto. A blended scent might offer a client the healing virtues of the single therapeutic scent as well as some hint of the marvelous attitude that kept Otto alive long past doctors' predictions.

Now, in taking a full scope of the possibilities of aromatherapy, one fact that becomes clear is that there are a myriad of different aromas, and even more when the possibilities of all the different blended combinations are considered. There are also a multitude of varying situations that may be remedied with the arts of the aromatherapist. Because of this, while some of us may expound the virtues of pure scents over blends, blends over single essentials, natural oils above synthetics, or synthetics above the natural, what we all seek is that which is effective. Therefore, perhaps the wisest precept to advocate is to keep an open mind and to address each situation as it needs be. If the cause calls for a blend, then so be it. If a pure single fragrance is the ideal approach, then by all means that is the way to go.

There is a lot of artistry in the process of blending the best-suited preparation for use in aromatherapy. Certainly, it tests the knowledge, expertise, instinct, and sensitivity of the practitioner. However, there is even greater artistry involved in choosing the right essential or combination of essentials for each individual situation—without regard to founding principles or schools of thought but with every consideration of the recipient of the benefits of the fragrance artistry.

Magickal Associations

In addition to the traditional practices of our ancestors, there are other criteria used as guidelines in the preparation of aromatherapy formulae. These are rooted in practices of long ago but they allow flexibility in the development of new blends and the advancement of the art. According to many of the ancient magick-al traditions, there are influences that permeate the universe, push-ing our lives this way and that, determining our fates. As natural forces ebb and flow, we are carried on the momentum of their courses. The function of magick, then, is to work with these forces; to captivate them and persuade them to lead us in a predetermined direction; to gain order and control in our lives.

There are many different areas of domination in which universal energies are perceived. Some magicians practice their art in accor-dance with the properties of the four great elements of creation—earth, air, fire, and water. In the beginning of time, before the advent of creation, some traditions perceive all the universe's ener-gy, the source of all life, as being embodied as a single power. As creation began to unfold, this oneness split into four distinct aspects, the four elements. Though each sprang from the same source, they have uniquely individual characteristics and different areas of domination. These differences will become foundational requirements when choosing the ideal essential oil or oil blend to utilize for a successful magickal operation.

There are some magical disciplines that recog-nize distinctly different influences in the days of the week, and ride the height of the proper day's influence to accomplish their magickal tasks. Some look to gods and goddesses of cultures ancient and modern. Others ride the power surges that rise and fall with the phases of the moon. Still others note the astrological planets and signs in approaching a magickal undertaking.

While there is one segment of aromatherapy practitioners who fancy themselves being of scientific mind and above the use of the trappings of folklore and so-called superstitious belief, these guidelines are as applicable today as they were in less "enlightened" times. Even the scientific mind will allow that the proof of a remedy lies in its effectiveness. No matter where its roots may lie, if the end product is something that is usable and effective, it remains above the challenges of the scientific community.

There is an old story about a mathematician who challenged the ability of a friend to walk across the room. He took the position that before making the journey, the friend would have to first cover half the distance, then, half the distance of that, and half again, and again, and again. There would always be some distance remaining that could be divided in half. Being less sophisticated in the ways of science and mathematics, the friend walked briskly to the other side of the room, kicked the wall, and said, "You're wrong, my friend!" The greatest of logic must give way in the face of physical reality; the governing factor in aromatherapy is not the individual practitioner's perception of it but the reality that it does work.

If the traditional oil associations do not fit well into the world in which you've become comfortable, change the names of the traditional categories or consider them temporary labels until the scientific community can discover the "real" reason that they work—but do try them. The final judgment of an oil mixture should be in its effectiveness. It matters little whether it is directed toward healing or magickal application. The only question should be "Does it work?"

While it can be truly said that there is no absolute right and wrong in preparing magickal aromatic blends, the knowledge and skill of the individual artisan can attain levels of better and best, less or more effective. As in healing aromatherapy, the instincts of the practitioner will play a major role in the fulfillment of the ultimate purpose. Armed with the knowledge of the innate properties and functions of each of the essential oils, the resulting blended fragrance can be finely tuned to suit any magickal endeavor.

The fragrance magician who works in conjunction with the traditional astrological disciplines must ingest a world of knowledge before settling down to the mastery of magickal aromatherapy. However, just as it is possible to perceive the influences traditionally associated in astrological science on several levels, one can enter into the ways of the aromatherapist in stages. While all of the energies of the astrological divisions may ultimately become invaluable tools of knowledge to the practicing magician, it is easier to embark on the magickal journey one step at a time.

In the beginning stages of learning fragrance magick, it is possible to begin working only elementally or only planetarily. It is possible to complete a successful magickal venture using only the basic knowledge of one or two levels of astrological association. As knowledge increases, presumably so will the effectiveness of the undertaking and the ease with which the essential blends are produced. It would be a mistake, and perhaps a bit irresponsible, to try to take in the whole of aromatherapy magick in a single sitting. However, given the patience and time to learn and grow and develop, the sincere student of the aromatic arts may attain to successes beyond what might have been thought possible. Entered into sincerely, and with a desire to expand the art to its furthest capabilities, these first steps become the beginning of a never-ending, always exciting adventure.

Male and Female

If we consider the many oils available that may be employed in a blend designed to a given purpose, the process of choosing the right oils in each specific endeavor may seem overwhelming. However, taken in steps, it becomes a much simpler procedure; essentially, a process of elimination. Initially, we will note the most general category: that of gender correspondence. Like much that exists in nature, oils innately have a female or male nature to them. Basically, the male scent is one that is more aggressive in its action, while the female scent is more passive. The male scent is more physical, and the female more emotional and intuitive. The importance of determining the gender characteristics of an aromatic substance is that it enables the aromatherapy magician to designate not only what effect the end combination of oils will have but in what way it will affect the subject of the rite.

Like the oriental principle of yin and yang, the manner in which an essential oil works may be characterized in one of two ways. There is the male and female, the active and passive, light and dark, practical and emotional, or the pragmatic and the imaginative. These seemingly opposite qualities play an important role in the fulfillment of magickal process.

In applying these general traits to the design of an oil blend, we need only consider the purpose of its application. If, for example, we are addressing a situation of hyperactivity, fear, or nervousness, we may employ a female scent. In the case of apathy, laziness, or anemia, we may turn to the male scents to balance the condition. In magickal workings, if we wish to enhance romantic feelings of love, a female oil may best suit our needs. The more aggressive feelings of passion could be better enhanced with a male scent.

In the case of a healing rite, for example—what exactly is the nature of the illness? If the subject suffers from lethargy, perhaps the interjection of a male, or aggressive, oil would be in order. For a raging fever, a female, or passive, oil may be more appropriate. Familiarity with the natural gender characteristics of the essential components of an oil blend will arm the practitioner with the ability to accomplish the task at hand as well as determine in what manner it is to be realized.

One of the basic magickal principles in discovering the duality in aromatherapy as well as that reflected in nature is the recognition and understanding of the reconciliation of opposites. The male and female natures have been referred to as seemingly opposite qualities. This is, in fact, by design. For in altering a situation through magickal application, very often all that we are doing is restoring a natural state of balance. We counterbalance an overabundance of female characteristics with male energies, and compensate for an overly male nature with the introduction of female forces.

Consider the images of a mother and father figure. Where a child might retreat to the mother figure for love, compassion, and security, the same child may seek out the father for protection, strength, and stability. Though different, the male and female approaches to the same situation are interrelated. In a rite of protection, the sense of security provided in the arms of the mother is no less valid than the feeling of solid shelter we find in the shadow of the strong father figure. There is a place for each expression of the same principle. The ideal approach is not determined by the gender of the magician or the subject or by any personal beliefs or preferences but by the nature of the specific situation. Specific problems demand specific remedies.

It is said that every male has a female side and every female, a masculine aspect to their being. This is a clue to the use of gender in magick. When all is right, when everything is stable in our lives, we have not achieved the ultimate of our masculine or feminine natures but have realized a comfortable balance between the two. Anytime we encounter a situation that creates conflict or negativity in our lives, it can be perceived as a falling-out of balance. If we restore that balance, the situation is remedied.

In another way of looking at the male and female aspects in all of nature, we might keep in mind the functioning of innate roles in reproduction. Male and female combine to bear new life. Likewise, in magickal workings, the restoration of balance in our life situations is akin to the union of the masculine and feminine principles. When the two work together as one, we witness a birth. In the case of magickal workings, the new birth is the change in the situation for which the magickal process has been undertaken.

In the appendix, a table of male and female essential oils has been included. Combined with magickal properties and other characteristics, this information will enable the practitioner of fragrance sorcery to determine to best scent or combination of scents for use in the specific magickal application.

Planets and Signs

Most magickal associations can be examined in basic terms of the astrological planets and signs of the zodiac. Each day of the week has an associated, or ruling, planet. The influences of the particular day are not unlike those of its planetary ruler. Monday, for instance, is ruled by Mercury. The winged messenger rules communication, intelligence, travel, writing, the conscious mind, and learning. These, then, are the same influences as would be ascribed to a day of the week. It is necessary only to know the station each planet takes on the weekly calendar to determine the influence of the day.

As for the planets themselves, there are nine that are generally accepted as the basis for astrological calculation and interpretation. They are the Sun, the Moon, Mercury, Venus, Mars, Neptune, Uranus, Saturn, and Jupiter. Some astrologers also note Pluto— although it had not yet been discovered at the time of the development of the astrological arts, it is sometimes acknowledged as a separate influence by modern-day astrologers. However, many consider this tenth planetary rulership of secondary significance. It is felt that, being small in comparison to the other spheres and the most distant, Pluto exerts only a minor influence.

The areas of rulership for each of the planets is very distinct. Each has its own dominion, its own area of influence. Each takes reign over specific traits of human existence, areas of social endeavor, and is even associated with specific parts of the human body. This could be valuable criteria to keep in mind when using essential oils for healing as well as magick.

The **Sun** is the planet of self-expression. It rules vitality, health, creativity, fatherhood, children, and self-empowerment. It is associated with the heart and the spinal column.

The **Moon** is an influence of the subconscious. It is the planet of instinctive response, emotion, imagination, psychic development, home, family, motherhood, and birth. The stomach, digestive system, and breasts (especially female) are under the Moon's control. The Sun and Moon are as the father and mother of the planetary influences. The Sun embraces the patriarchal principle, and the Moon is the matriarchal.

Intellect, perception, wisdom, learning, communication, and travel are within the kingdom of **Mercury**. The respiratory system and the thyroid gland are also within Mercury's reign.

The ways of love and union are watched over by **Venus**. In her dominion, romance and the language of romance thrives. Venus is ruler of love, partnership, poetry, beauty, fertility, and the arts. She also rules the lower back, the throat, and the kidneys.

Mars, the warrior planet, takes control over passion, aggression, determination, and initiative. The muscles, the blood, and the reproductive systems are his domain. Similar to the Sun and Moon, Mars and Venus may be viewed as a couple. Mars reflects all that is masculine and Venus is the planet of feminine virtue.

Business, knowledge, and philosophy are under the controlling
hand of **Jupiter**. Religion, education, publication, and good
fortune are also within Jupiter's sphere of influence. The
liver and the pituitary gland belong to his kingdom.

Saturn is an influence of containment, restriction, inhibition,
intolerance, rigidity, old age, perseverance, and slow change.
Not surprisingly, the parts of the body under the hand of
Saturn are those associated with slowing down—those that
make themselves known with old age. Saturn rules the gall
bladder, restriction in the joints, bones, teeth, skin, and the
spleen. With its associations with old age also comes an
awareness of death and dying, of that which is unseen and
unknown. Therefore, there are connections with Saturn to
deep religion and the occult.

The twin planets of Uranus and Neptune carry us beyond the
reaches of the mundane, beyond what may be considered normal
and acceptable. While in one sense they may be considered to rule
the adventurer, in another they could be considered to rule those
who have slipped over the edge of reality and beyond the reaches
of rational thought and action.

Uranus is the planet of research, science, and development. It
takes rulership over science, electronics, journeys in outer
space, radio, television, video, and science fiction. It is also
associated with the circulation, nervous disorders, and with
sexual perversion and deviations.

Neptune is ruler of drugs and poisons, of hospitals, prisons,
and other institutions. It is the king of religious and artistic
inspiration and, as such, may sometimes flirt with obsession.
More than any other planet, Neptune takes dominion over
the nerves.

Finally, we approach the kingdom of **Pluto**—the last of the honored planetary realms. Pluto is associated with beginnings and endings, with death and regeneration. It is also connected, like Mars, to the reproductive organs. In some ways, it could be considered a marriage of the influences of Mars and Saturn. While its influence has the aggressive, active thrust of Mars, it may be drawn in the direction of the darker pursuits of Saturn.

Further defining the planets are the signs of the zodiac. Each of the twelve signs is ruled by a governing planetary body. These appear below, along with their planetary ruler. The influence of the associated planet to each sign is clearly apparent in the type of characteristics traditionally associated with each sign.

Aries (Mars)	Assertive, adventurous, courageous
Taurus (Venus)	Affectionate, warm, trustworthy, reliable, patient, possessive, solid
Gemini (Mercury)	Communicative, adaptable, versatile, intellectual, spontaneous
Cancer (Moon)	Motherly, empathetic, protective, imaginative, caring; the sign of the homemaker
Leo (Sun)	Proud, creative, powerful, enthusiastic
Virgo (Mercury)	Analytical, discriminating, modest
Libra (Venus)	Artistic, harmonious, romantic, diplomatic
Scorpio (Mars/Pluto)	Passionate, intense, dramatic, powerful, determined, purposeful
Sagittarius (Jupiter)	Sincere, open, optimistic, philosophical, dependable

Capricorn (Saturn)	Calculated, ambitious, careful, disciplined
Aquarius (Uranus)	Progressive, humanitarian, intellectual, inventive, independent, adventurous
Pisces (Neptune)	Emotional, impressionable, intuitive, receptive

It should be noted that while there are specific general characteristics that are embodied by each of the astrological signs, these may be expressed in a positive or a negative manner. For example, strength may be expressed as bullying behavior, independence as contrariness, or receptiveness as weakness of will. Herein lies the beauty of the magick of fragrance. Blending different scents enables us to fine-tune the overall result of the working influence. The entire process becomes a finer, more precisely directed art. It is lifted from the realm of hit and miss and effectiveness is increased significantly.

Elemental Association

To the astrologer, the signs are seen as being grouped by elemental association. The specific rulerships of the signs offer some insight into the more widely encompassing associations of elemental influence. Generally, the four cardinal elements can be divided into their own areas of control. It can be readily seen how the planets and signs fit into these general categories of influence.

The four elements are earth, air, fire, and water.

Earth includes the zodiac signs of Taurus, Virgo, and Capricorn. Earth exerts influence on material possessions, money, business, deep strength, reason, justice, understanding, and stability.

The element of **air** is home to Gemini, Libra, and Aquarius. This is the sphere of travel, communication, movement, learning, writing, faith, intuition, and knowledge.

Fire is host to Aries, Leo, and Sagittarius. Fire speaks of passion, determination, war, aggression, conflict, hope, and courage.

The final elemental realm of **water** is the land of Cancer, Scorpio, and Pisces. Water is the realm of love, emotion, charity, beauty, spirituality, psychic development, intuition, and compassion.

Each scent can be placed in general associations with the ancient elements of earth, air, fire, or water. In many cases, a scent—while exemplifying the virtues of a particular element very strongly—may have hints of an undertone, or a secondary association, with another of the elements.

Accordingly, to calm irrational behavior, an **earth oil** may be a major component of a blend. Magickally, these oils may be used to address physical stability and well-being— for example, material gain, securing a job, or promoting justice in court.

Air oils may be enlisted in the production of an essential blend aimed at promoting easy breathing, helping to clear confusion, or enhancing learning pursuits for the active student.

In addressing phobias, enhancing passion, or raising the energy level, **fire oils** may be brought into play. This example also brings to light a situation in which the virtues of more than one element are essential. In relieving irrational fears, for example, we may wish to employ the virtue of courage that a fire oil will afford us. However, because of the virtue of increasing energy, an oil corresponding to fire may actually have the effect of feeding the fear and worsening the condition. Therefore, it is wise to temper the fire with earth. The overall result is that we may gain courage from the fire element while maintaining stability and control with the element of earth.

The virtues of the water element in **water oils** may be used to increase fluidity, as in cases of poor circulation, or may be used to enhance romantic love and increase psychic development.

Gods and Goddesses

One of the methods of completing a successful operation of magick is to enlist the aid of divine forces. In addition to their inherent properties, many essential oils take on a special association with a particular god or goddess from the mythology of different cultures. The use of a scent sacred to the particular divinity invoked for a rite does honor to the divine personage and may be an excellent way to gain his or her favor over the magickal quest. The same principle of seeking the favor of outside agents in magick may apply equally in the case of demigods, cultural heroes, and honored ancestors.

Some hint of which scent is sacred to which divinity may be gained from the traditional legends from which we remember the adventures of the divine beings. This is especially true of the ancient Greek and Roman divinities. In fact, in these cases, many of the associations are easily discerned, for many of the source plants of essential oils are derived from the ancient languages of these cultures and, in translation, speak of the divine being to whom they have special significance.

Consider, for instance, the herb angelica. During the middle ages, when the line of definition between medicine and magick was indistinct, angelica was employed as the first line of defense against the black plague. Was its use rooted in its curative properties or in seeking the blessings of the angels, as its name suggests? Rose, a flower and scent beloved of many cultures, is sacred to both the Greek goddess of flowers, Chloris, and her Roman equivalent, Flora. Water lily carries a scientific name of Nymphaea. Originally from the Greek, this name suggests that the lily may be a fragrance sacred to the water nymphs of mythology. The violet is said to have originated from the tears of the goddess Io, beloved of Zeus, the father of the Greek gods. It is reasonable to assume that this fragrance might gain the goddess' attention if offered to her honor. Iris is the Greek word for rainbow, and is also the name of the goddess of the rainbow. Bay laurel, according to legend, began as the nymph Daphne. Apollo so loved the nymph that a waft of her scent may gain the gift of his divine assistance in works of magick.

For lack of a specific fable that indicates an association of a scent with a particular divinity, there are some more general principles for honoring the gods and goddesses whose favor we seek. Just as the rose is sacred to the goddesses of flowers, it is a favored fragrance among many of the goddesses of myth. Pine, often associated with the Greek god Pan, is a likely scent to offer many of the male divinities, particularly those who dwell among the creatures of the forest. Oak, the king of trees, is a fitting scent for the kings of gods in many cultures. It might be a suitable offering to Zeus, Woden, or Jupiter.

Civet, originally derived from feline secretions, could be used to the glory of the Egyptian cat goddess, Bast. Earthy fragrances— flowers, grasses, and herbs—could be a fitting tribute to Demeter or any of the many other earth goddesses.

Frankincense and myrrh, while designated as proper offerings to the Christ child in well-known biblical legends, are scents that have been revered throughout many cultures. These sacred fragrances would be right at home in many temples and churches regardless of religious doctrine, sect, or tradition. These ancient aromatics have been a staple in religious rite and magickal ceremony throughout the ages of man, and have survived the rise and fall of many great cultures.

Eastern divinities may favor the aromas that are tied to Eastern culture. Jasmine, sandalwood, lotus, and Chinese musk could be employed for rites of the oriental deities. Sage would be a fitting tribute to the gods and goddesses of American Indian mythology, and patchouli a proper scent for the deities of India.

In many cases, the sagas of deities and heroes that survive in the legendry and folklore of different cultures will dictate the preferences of the various gods and goddesses. There are, however, some catch-all guidelines in choosing a proper scent for religious and magickal use. In general, the floral scents are thought to be more female in nature and pleasing to most goddesses. The more woodsy fragrances are considered more masculine and, therefore, suitable offerings to the male deities. Also, the associated planets of the scents can act as a guideline to determine which essential oil would be most proper and fitting to a particular deity. Looking to the Roman gods and goddesses from which the planets take their names, we find that they each have corresponding deities in other cultures. Jupiter, for example, is the strong father god. In his nature, he is not unlike Zeus of Greek mythology, Woden of Norse legend, or the Dagda of the Celtic culture. Venus is a spiritual sister of Aphrodite, Freya, and Bridget. There are many crossovers between cultures. And though the Greek and Roman traditions are the most universally remembered, other cultures have not neglected the realms of the traditional deities though they may appear in different form, their praises sung in different tongues, and their names be other than what is recorded in the classical mythology. And as they share a common nature and a common soul, the deities of many cultures can share the tribute of a shared essential fragrance.

Cultural Considerations

Some fragrances are rooted deeply into a particular culture or a particular magickal tradition. While some examples of this may be seen through connections to various gods and goddesses or through the mythology and folklore of a specific country or geographic area, others that are commonplace in certain practices may never appear in the local legendry. These scents gain a place of extreme importance within their designated cultures through popular usage.

Consider, for example, the American capital of voodoo practice—New Orleans. Along with visions of spiritism and Mardi Gras, one might imagine the sweet fragrance of magnolias. This scent appears in many of the traditional love oils that originate in New Orleans. This scent was made popular by the women who earned their livings in the New Orleans brothels in the 1800s. Not surprisingly, it is an especially commonplace ingredient in magickal formulas directed toward the arousal of passions in men.

If we direct our thoughts to the Caribbean islands, we may think about the smell of coconuts, bananas, and limes. It's no wonder that the use of limes in essential form or in raw fruit appears in many of the Caribbean rites of Santería magick.

Patchouli is a popular scent in Mexico. Sage is common among the magickal practices of Native American shamans. Vanilla is a magickal staple of African practices. In the Orient, willow is the scent of friendship, renewal, perseverance, and humility, while thyme, to the ancient Greeks, symbolizes courage.

Buddhists favor sandalwood as an incense to be burned during funeral rites. This is the continuation of a popular usage established in ancient times. It is interesting to note that sandalwood originates from India and China, two of the great lands that are home to Buddhist practice.

Muguet is an essential oil produced from a certain species of lily of the valley that grows only in a small area in France. It is no wonder that this scent was favored as a highly valued scent by exclusive French perfumers. Its use in magickal formulas may also originate specifically from France. Although it is not a common ingredient to most blenders of magickal scents, those who know how to use it find it invaluable.

Considerations of popular usage are also imperative to the creation of appropriate scents for specific magickal purposes. As an example, there was a request submitted to me for a specifically Celtic oil for use in rituals of Celtic-based pagan practice. The way I created this was to find ingredients that suited the purpose of enhancing ritual work but were also native to the lands that were inhabited by the old Celts. There were two different formulas that were developed out of this research. Each is very specifically for use in Celtic ritual. Each has a specific purpose, and each is highly effective.

In addition to capturing the magickal properties of a given scent, it is possible to utilize its origin and the history of its popular usage. To capture specific properties or isolated virtues in preparing a magickal blend is but one level of working. Through careful study and consideration it is possible to capture the nature of an entire culture or race of people within a blended formula. The resulting fragrance is the embodiment of the mentality, heart, and soul of a society, or group mind of a people. It is the essence of their thoughts and beliefs and approach to spirit, virtue, and everyday living.

Without intending to undervalue the blending of magickal essentials by traditional properties and effect, it should be noted that there are different ways to approach the magickal blend. In looking to the religious, mythological, cultural, and social aspects of scent, we are working the magick at its deepest, most secret heart of truth. We are pushing quality to its maximum extent and creating the most effective combinations possible. On one level, it could be said that this full scope of recognition allows us to excel in the art of essential magick. On another, considering the knowledge of the hidden magickal arts as a divine gift, we do the greatest possible honor to the gods and goddesses who are our benefactors in granting us access to this arcane knowledge. The more attentive we are to the depth of our art, the greater the tribute we offer for this gift.

These are general classifications of influences. Between the overview of properties offered in this chapter and the tables included in the appendix, even a novice aromatherapist should be able to understand the basic workings of the fragrance arts. There are so many formulas included in this writing that have been field tested and proven in effectiveness that, if the general blending instructions are followed, the result should be an effective blend. The more advanced practitioner will be able to enhance the effectiveness of his or her blends by virtue of developed knowledge and experience. But even newcomers to the art of aromatherapy should experience some significant successes with the included blends.

ragrance in Use

A Case Study in Blending

While most of the basic principles have been addressed within the body of this text, there is still the business of translating these concepts into reality. Between the introduction of the workings of aromatherapy, the charts and tables of magickal influences, the narration of possible application, and the example formulas, there is a solid basis for a beginning or expansion

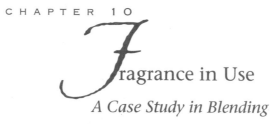

of an aromatherapy practice. However, now we must take these bits and pieces and put them all together. It is no small endeavor. In fact, it might be likened to the task of the criminal investigator, who must take all the clues, all the tidbits of evidence, all the observations, and even the hearsay, and come to a probable re-creation of events to solve a mystery. We are pouring all these little bits of foundational material into a great funnel and attempting to produce a perfect aromatic oil blend for a given situation.

In order to clearly illustrate the process, we will again resort to examples. However, in this case, we will compare similarly directed magickal blends to one another to define the subtleties of difference between them. In analyzing the composition of these examples, it may help to clarify the process of producing oil blends.

In this case, we will use two original formulas. Both are love oils. However, they are directed along the lines of different intentions. "Love's Heart" is a blend that is applied toward the enhancement of romantic love. "Love's Passion" is used to develop the more physical expressions of emotional arousal.

The general formulae are as follows:

Love's Heart

rose (MA)
gardenia (mi)
lavender (mi)

Love's Passion

jasmine (MA)
rose (MA)
sandalwood (MA)
patchouli (MA)
camphor! (T)

As discussed previously, there are three general categories of ingredients in a blend—the major ingredients (MA), the minor ingredients (mi), and the trace elements (T). Just to recall what we have discussed previously, the major influences would appear in the blend in the greatest quantity, the minor influences are in evidence to a lesser degree, and the trace elements are included in very small amounts—only a drop, or a few drops. Scanning the formulae for these two oil blends side by side, the first obvious difference is that Love's Heart does not utilize the trace element, and Love's Passion has no minor influences. This offers some hint as to the workings of each blend and some indication of the effects of trace elements and minor influences. But let's pick apart the formulae in some detail to see the hows and whys of their compositions.

Beginning with Love's Heart, the major influence lies in the properties of the rose oil. Looking at the background information already given regarding rose, we uncover many elements that show clear cause for its inclusion in the above blend. Rose is an oil sacred to Venus, the Roman goddess of love and beauty. Likewise, it is a special scent to Aphrodite, the Greek counterpart of Venus. Its magickal properties include matters of love as well as peace and harmony, elements necessary to creating an atmosphere of romance. Among others of its therapeutic properties, rose oil is known for its aphrodisiac properties. It is used in the treatment of frigidity and impotence. Thus, it has a similar effect on both male and female. Romantic love most decidedly is a venture of sharing. Elemental jurisdiction gives the scent of rose to earth—the element of stability, fertility, and stabilization. It is a fragrance of Libra and Cancer. Libra's key words are beauty and creativity. Cancer is the nurturing influence of home life. The combination of these influences sets the stage for romance, for soft creative beauty, for love.

Minor influences in Love's Heart are gardenia and lavender. Gardenia emphasizes the properties of water, Libra, and Venus. Its magickal properties emphasize love, peace, and spirituality—again, bringing out the softer side of love, the shared emotion and spirit, the romance. Lavender adds a touch of the intellectual. It is associated with air, Mercury, and the signs of Gemini and Virgo. These influences bring thoughtfulness to the union. Gemini and Virgo underscore the properties of beauty and creativity, or care and softness. Combined with the love influence of rose, these minor influences create a softness, developing the beautiful, caring, romantic side of an emotional bond. Lavender also helps to instill trust. It is used therapeutically to relieve feelings of fear and suspicion. The soft, emotional, thoughtful side of love is the essence of romance. This carefully selected trio of ingredients result in a blend that not only addresses the prospect of love but carries it along a specifically chosen direction.

Love's Passion, on the other hand, is designed to address the more fiery, explosive aspect of love. It does not address the love that is borne of the mind and soul but rather of the passionate heart and the hot blood. The four major ingredients in this blend are rose, jasmine, sandalwood, and patchouli. Part of the business of arousing the passions is to set the stage. By capturing the love properties of rose, we place ourselves in the proper arena in which to raise the fury of love's passion. Jasmine is water/earth, Taurus/ Cancer, and Jupiter/Moon. To the stabilizing influence of earth, we add the emotional properties of the element of water. To the nurturing properties of Cancer, we add the more aggressive properties of Taurus. Jupiter is a "take control" influence, while the Moon touches the unconscious mind—the realm in which the instincts that give way to the arousal of sexual desire lay waiting. Patchouli is under the influence of earth, Taurus/Capricorn, and Saturn. While some of these influences enhance the properties that already are in evidence through the other essential ingredients, others bring out different properties. The influence of Capricorn adds a touch of fire to the effect of our blend. It is the essence of arousal. Saturn is used therapeutically to lift inhibitions. It is, therefore, a perfect influence to allow the lovers to give way to passion. Sandalwood is earth/water, Jupiter/Neptune, and Cancer/Pisces. Again, many of the previously stated influences are enhanced. However, sandalwood also brings some new properties to the blend. The addition of Neptune addresses depth. It arouses the depth of emotion. The influence of Pisces has a similar effect. Again, it reaches down deep where free expression and abandonment of restrictive inhibitions dwell. Sandalwood also parallels the odor of the human sex hormone, alpha androsterole. There is little question that this will directly address that aspect of love we wish to develop. This works quite directly on the instincts of passionate love.

Finally, there is the inclusion of camphor as a trace element in the Love's Passion blend. The associations of camphor are water, Cancer, and the Moon. All of these influences have already been addressed in other ingredients. This is where it becomes important to understand the action of the trace element on the overall effect of the blend. Those who have studied the workings of homeopathy are familiar with the principle that more is less. In order to strengthen a homeopathic remedy, it is decreased in strength. Homeopathy uses catalysts to spur on the body's own natural mechanisms of reaction. While the practice of homeopathy is involved, to a large extent, in the awakening of the immune system in the treatment of disorders, aromatherapy may be used in a parallel way to arouse the inborn systems of instinctual response.

Camphor is used therapeutically as a tonic to arouse energy. It can be used as a kind of smelling salt. With its piercing aroma, it has some shock value. It acts as a call to arms for body and mind. Magickally, it can be used to awaken past lives. Again, it reaches deep inside the individual and shakes loose the things that are buried or inhibited. Its inclusion in this formula is to awaken the deepest seeds of passion, to shake loose the restrictions of social prejudicial behavior, and to touch the base instincts that lie dormant in all of us.

Again, to relate its effect to homeopathy, there are other parallels. Homeopathy, in its remedies, uses trace amounts of poisons—elements that, if introduced to the body in greater amounts, would cause sickness or death. The trace elements included in many aromatherapy blends are those that are most highly irritating. Some of the prime candidates for use as trace elements are:

anise, cayenne, cinnamon, citronella, clove, frankincense, lemon, lemongrass, lemon verbena, myrrh, oakmoss, orange, peppermint, wintergreen

Not all of these trace oils are addressed specifically in the text of this presentation because they are not main staples of my own personal selection of oils. However, because they are readily available, and because I do heartily encourage responsible experimentation, they are included here with the warning that they may act as major irritants (and they are marked accordingly in the text with an exclamation [!] mark). Responsible aromatherapy demands the exercise of caution and careful consideration.

Hopefully, these sample blends will illuminate some of the subtleties that are encountered in the art of magickal aromatherapy. It is possible to specifically direct the effect of a magickal blend to a very precise purpose, to respond to an individual situation, a finely tuned purpose, an exact need. Of course, expertise in the art of producing aromatic blends is elevated through the continued development of knowledge, experience, and inspiration. The information revealed within these pages is designed to form a stable and broad foundation from which to strive for increase and expansion.

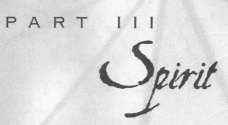

PART III

Spirit

*Essences
of
Aromatherapy*

CHAPTER 11

Therapeutic Blends

With the general formulae in place, we can look into specific combinations of essentials for various purposes. Although in most cases the expertise and creative healing ability of the individual aromatherapist is encouraged in adapting the specific remedy to the needs of the client, for the purpose of example, precise ratios will be used in the introductory blends that follow.

These are but a sampling of the many possible therapeutic blends that can be produced and applied by the aromatherapist. Through variation of component essentials and specific amounts within each formula, the possible remedies available to the fragrance artisan is limitless. The effectiveness of any given blend is bound only by the practical expertise and instinctive artistry of the individual practitioner. These are but the first tiny steps into a vast universe teeming with natural wonders.

Respiratory Ailments

3	parts pine	3	parts spearmint
3	parts lavender	2	parts rosemary!
1¾	parts eucalyptus	2	parts clove!
1¾	parts lemon!	1	part lime
½	part lime	1	part lavender

4	parts clove!	3	parts rosemary!
2	parts cypress	3	parts clove!
2	parts pine	2	parts pine
1	part lemon!	1	part orange!

Recommended application: Inhalant (use in oil burner or with vaporizer will be most effective)

Relief of Stress

4½	parts lavender	5	parts sandalwood
4½	parts orange!	2	parts lavender
2	parts pine		

5	parts lemon verbena!	5	parts vetivert
4	parts galangal	2	parts cinnamon!
2	parts bay		

Recommended application: Bath, spray, or inhalant (be careful of irritant oils!)

Energy

6	parts lime	3	parts lemon!
2	parts peppermint!	3	parts cypress
1	part orange!	3	parts clove!

4	parts ylang ylang	3	parts frankincense!
2	parts galangal	3	parts galangal
1½	parts patchouli	3	parts orange!
1½	parts lime		

Recommended application: Bath, inhalant

Sore Muscles

3	parts ylang ylang	3	parts bay
3	parts galangal	2	parts rosemary!
1½	parts clove!	2	parts eucalyptus
1½	parts rosemary!	2	parts ylang ylang

2	parts cinnamon!	3½	parts galangal
2	parts rose	2	parts cinnamon!
1¾	parts juniper berry	1¾	parts clove!
1¾	parts lavender	1¾	parts bay
1½	parts wintergreen!		

Recommended application: Bath, massage (be careful of irritant oils!)

Insomnia

2½	parts benzoin	3	parts lavender
1½	parts bay	2	parts rose
1¾	parts cedar	2	parts bergamot!
1¾	parts sandalwood	2	parts bay
1½	parts lemon!		

3½	parts orange!	2½	parts pine
1¾	parts galangal	2½	orange!
1¾	parts cedar	2½	parts lavender
1½	parts bay	1½	parts galangal

Recommended application: Inhalant (through oil burner or vaporizer while settling down to sleep)

_A_dvanced Therapeutic Blends

There are, as would be expected, a limitless number of possible combinations of fragrant blends. Because of space restrictions, many of the possible therapeutic formulas have been omitted. Those that have been included, however, comprise a solid basis for a sound therapeutic practice in aromatherapy.

The blends that are included here are of two basic types. Some have been taken from the scent-healing practices of others. Of these, only the ones that are based in sound aromatherapy principles have been listed. The main criteria for those presented here is that the ingredients can be analyzed in accordance with accepted foundational scent associations, and the basis easily understood for each ingredient's inclusion in the formula.

The second type of formula included is that of personal design. These blends have been tried in actual practice and have proven themselves to be well worth including in an arsenal of therapeutic remedies.

Again, it should be emphasized that the formulae included in these pages are written in a loose, non-stringent manner. The individual creativity and expertise of the practitioner is encouraged. The continued awareness of the need to address each client and each situation in the light of its own merit is also encouraged. The non-specific presentation of ingredient amounts should help to maximize the benefit of these all-important considerations. Yet the quality of the guidelines should serve well in the hands of the thinking practitioner.

For easier reference, the therapeutic blends have been divided into five different sections. Each section addresses the type of condition to be treated, as dictated by the bodily functions that it deals with. This should make finding specific blends far easier as it becomes necessary to refer back to them. Recommended methods of application have also been included for each fragrant blend. These are by no means hard and fast rules, but merely suggestions. As always, creativity is encouraged. Still, it may be helpful to know what type of transmittal systems have already proven effective in actual practice for specific blends.

Life's Substance (The Body)

Muscle Relaxers

cedarwood (MA)
cypress (MA)
lavender (MA)
lemon verbena! (mi)

Recommended application: Bath

sandalwood (MA)
cypress (MA)
lavender (mi)
clove! (T)
cinnamon! (T)

Recommended application: Bath

Soothe Aching Muscles

orange! (MA)
lavender (MA)
cinnamon! (T)
clove! (T)

Recommended application: Bath

cypress (MA)
cinnamon! (mi)
rose (mi)
lemon! (T)

Recommended application: Bath

Soothe Aching Muscles, continued

rose (MA)
ylang ylang (MA)
spearmint (mi)
lavender (T)

Recommended application: Bath, massage

galangal (MA)
bay (MA)
cinnamon! (T)
clove! (T)

Recommended application: Local massage

rose (MA)
eucalyptus (MA)
pine (MA)

Recommended application: Local massage

rosemary! (MA)
lavender (MA)
galangal (mi)
clove! (T)

Recommended application: Local massage

pine (MA)
benzoin (mi)
galangal (mi)
cypress (mi)
rosemary! (mi)
juniper (T)
cedarwood (T)

Recommended application: Bath, massage

Increase Strength and Endurance

galangal (MA)
peppermint! (MA)
lemon! (mi)
bay (mi)

Recommended application: General massage

orange! (MA)
peppermint! (MA)
rose (MA)
eucalyptus (mi)
lime (mi)
galangal (T)

Recommended application: General massage

Sprains

cypress (MA)
rose (MA)
lemon verbena! (MA)

Recommended application: Local massage

lavender (MA)
galangal (MA)
peppermint! (mi)

Recommended application: Local massage

Fat Reduction

lemon! (MA)
juniper (MA)
lavender (MA)

Recommended application: Local and general massage

patchouli (MA)
lemon! (MA)

Recommended application: Local and general massage

Skin Inflammations, Acne

bergamot! (MA)
sandalwood (MA)
lavender (mi)

> **Recommended application:** Local

bergamot! (MA)
juniper (MA)
cedarwood (mi)
camphor! (T)

> **Recommended application:** Direct inhalation, local massage

Appendicitis

lavender (MA)

> **Recommended application:** Bath, local massage (**Please note:** This is for temporary relief **only**! *See a qualified medical practitioner.*)

Bruises

lavender (MA)
orange! (MA)
rosemary! (MA)
rose (MA)
camphor! (T)
eucalyptus (T)

> **Recommended application:** Local

rose (MA)
lavender (MA)
sandalwood (MA)
frankincense! (MA)

> **Recommended application:** Direct or indirect inhalation, bath, full body or local massage

Reduce Perspiration

cypress (MA)
rosemary! (mi)
lavender (mi)

Recommended application: Bath

Ease Upset Stomach and Promote Digestion

galangal (MA)
bay (MA)
spearmint (mi)
wintergreen! (T)

Recommended Application: Direct or indirect inhalation,
bath, local massage

Relief of the Pain of Arthritis and Rheumatism

galangal (MA)
juniper (MA)
rosemary! (mi)
lemon verbena! (mi)
cedarwood (T)

Recommended application: Bath, massage

Abscess

bergamot! (MA)
lavender (MA)

Recommended application: Direct
inhalation, local massage

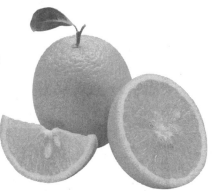

Life's Breath

Congestion Due to Allergies

orange! (MA)
rose (MA)
benzoin (mi)
peppermint! (mi)
eucalyptus (T)

Recommended application: Bath, direct or indirect inhalation

Head Colds

eucalyptus (MA)
peppermint! (T)
bay (T)

Recommended application: Direct or indirect inhalation

orange! (MA)
rosemary! (mi)
wintergreen! (T)
camphor! (T)
eucalyptus (T)

Recommended application: Direct or indirect inhalation

Bronchitis

bergamot! (MA)
eucalyptus (MA)
sandalwood (MA)

Recommended application: Direct or indirect inhalation

lemon! (MA)
sandalwood (MA)
lavender (mi)
camphor! (T)

Recommended application: Direct or indirect inhalation

Asthma

lavender (MA)
lily of the valley (MA)
orange! (MA)
benzoin (mi)
eucalyptus (T)

> **Recommended application:** Direct or indirect inhalation

Lung Disorders (Especially Emphysema)

eucalyptus (MA)

> **Recommended application:** Direct inhalation

Cough

benzoin (MA)
galangal (MA)
frankincense! (MA)
jasmine (MA)
peppermint! (T)
eucalyptus (T)

> **Recommended application:** Direct or indirect inhalation

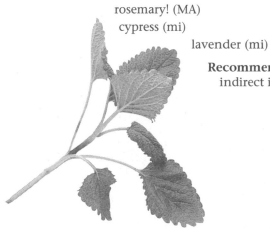

rosemary! (MA)
cypress (mi)
lavender (mi)

> **Recommended application:** Direct or indirect inhalation

General Relief of Breathing Difficulties

pine (MA)
rosemary! (MA)
cypress (MA)
camphor! (T)

Recommended application: Direct or indirect inhalation, bath

camphor! (MA)
eucalyptus (MA)
peppermint! (MA)

Recommended application: Direct or indirect inhalation, bath

rosemary! (MA)
rose (MA)
pine (mi)
bay (mi)
lime (mi)
cedarwood (T)

Recommended application: Indirect inhalation

Headache or Migraine (Especially Due to Congestion)

lavender (MA)
orange! (MA)
peppermint! (mi)
bay (T)

Recommended application: Direct inhalation,
bath, local massage

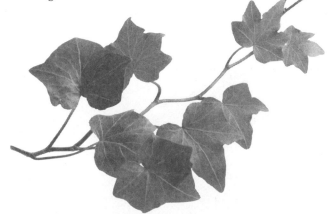

Life's Blood

Stop Bleeding

cypress (MA)
rose (MA)
lemon! (mi)

Recommended application: Direct inhalation

Blood Purifier

rose (MA)
juniper (MA)
rosemary! (mi)
eucalyptus (T)

Recommended application: Bath, direct or indirect inhalation

Stop Excessive Blood Loss

frankincense! (MA)
rose (MA)
cypress (mi)
cinnamon! (T)

Recommended application: Bath, direct or indirect inhalation

Build Up Blood

lemon! (MA)
galangal (MA)
rosemary! (MA)

Recommended application: Bath, direct or indirect inhalation, massage

Lower Blood Pressure

lavender (MA)
orange! (mi)
ylang ylang (mi)

Recommended application: Bath, indirect inhalation, massage

∽ *Raise Blood Pressure*

jasmine (MA)
rosemary! (mi)
pine (mi)

>**Recommended application:** Bath, direct or indirect inhalation, massage

∽ *Stimulate Circulation*

pine (MA)
rosemary! (MA)
bay (mi)
cinnamon! (T)
camphor! (T)

>**Recommended application:** Bath, direct inhalation, massage, local application (when appropriate)

Love in Life

∽ *Aphrodisiacs*

rose (MA)
sandalwood (MA)
jasmine (mi)

>**Recommended application:** Indirect inhalation, bath, massage

patchouli (MA)
musk (MA)
sandalwood (MA)
cinnamon! (T)

>**Recommended application:** Indirect inhalation

ylang ylang (MA)
ambergris (MA)
jasmine (mi)

>**Recommended application:** Indirect inhalation, bath

Impotence

rosemary! (MA)
jasmine (MA)
juniper (mi)
sandalwood (mi)

   Recommended application: Bath, massage, indirect inhalation

patchouli (MA)
musk (MA)
ambergris (mi)
muguet (T)

   Recommended application: Bath, indirect inhalation, massage

Sexually Transmitted Diseases

bergamot! (MA)
cedarwood (MA)
sandalwood (mi)
eucalyptus (T)

   Recommended application: Bath

Sterility

rose (MA)
orange! (mi)

   Recommended application: Bath

Painful Menstruation

rosemary! (MA)
cypress (MA)
jasmine (MA)
galangal (mi)
peppermint! (T)

   Recommended application: Bath, direct inhalation

⁀ *Premenstrual Syndrome (P.M.S.)*

bergamot! (MA)
rosemary! (MA)
orange! (MA)
ylang ylang (mi)

> **Recommended application:** Bath, direct or indirect inhalation

⁀ *Childbirth*

jasmine (MA)
lavender (mi)
rose (mi)

> **Recommended application:** Bath, direct or indirect inhalation

Mind and Spirit

⁀ *Ease Depression*

jasmine (MA)
lavender (MA)
orange! (MA)
oakmoss! (mi)
pine (mi)

> **Recommended application:**
> Direct or indirect inhalation,
> bath, massage

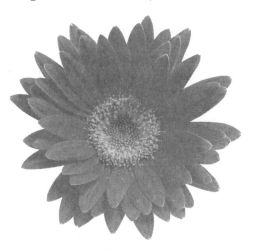

orange! (MA)
jasmine (MA)
lemon! (MA)

> **Recommended application:** Direct or indirect inhalation, bath, massage

bay (MA)
rose (MA)
jasmine (MA)
frankincense! (mi)
bergamot! (mi)
peppermint! (T)
ylang ylang (T)

> **Recommended application:** Bath, direct or indirect inhalation

Anxiety Relief

orange! (MA)
bergamot! (mi)
jasmine (mi)
spikenard (mi)
cedarwood (mi)
apple (T)
camphor! (T)

Recommended application: Direct inhalation

ylang ylang (MA)
orange! (MA)
pine (MA)

Recommended application: Direct or indirect inhalation,
bath, massage

cedarwood (MA)
lemon! (MA)
orange! (MA)

Recommended application: Direct inhalation, bath, massage

lavender (MA)
patchouli (MA)
orange! (MA)
pine (mi)
rosemary! (mi)

Recommended application: Direct or indirect inhalation

patchouli (MA)
rose (MA)
sandalwood (MA)
ylang ylang (MA)
benzoin (T)

Recommended application: Bath, direct or indirect inhalation

Ease Fear

juniper (MA)
lemon verbena! (MA)
spikenard (MA)
vetivert (MA)

Recommended application: Direct or indirect inhalation, massage

Impatience

frankincense! (MA)
lily of the valley (MA)
vanilla (MA)
lemon! (mi)
lemon verbena! (mi)

Recommended application: Direct inhalation, bath, massage

Mental Clarity

sandalwood (MA)
lavender (mi)
pine (mi)
musk (mi)
cinnamon! (T)

Recommended application: Direct or indirect inhalation

rose (MA)
lily of the valley (MA)
lavender (mi)
violet (mi)

Recommended application: Direct inhalation

Increased Communication

frankincense! (MA)
rosemary! (MA)
sandalwood (MA)

Recommended application: Direct inhalation, bath, massage

ylang ylang (MA)
pine (MA)
frankincense! (MA)

Recommended application: Direct inhalation, massage

Balancing

lemon! (MA)
orange! (MA)
lavender (MA)
myrrh! (MA)
clove! (T)

Recommended application: Direct inhalation, bath

Increased Concentration

myrrh! (MA)
violet (mi)
cinnamon! (T)

Recommended application: Direct inhalation

Courage

jasmine (MA)
pine (mi)
bay (T)
clove! (T)

Recommended application: Direct inhalation, bath

Increase Insights (and Foresight)

musk (MA)
ambergris (mi)
vetivert (mi)
violet (mi)
lilac (mi)

Recommended application: Direct or indirect inhalation

Dreams and Visions

magnolia (MA)
mimosa (MA)
orange! (MA)
violet (MA)

Recommended application: Bath, massage

⟿ Enhance Imagination

sandalwood (MA)
musk (mi)
galangal (mi)
cinnamon! (T)
clove! (T)

Recommended application: Direct or indirect inhalation

⟿ Promote More Social Behavior

carnation (MA)
gardenia (mi)
bergamot! (mi)
elderberry (mi)

Recommended application: Direct or indirect inhalation, bath

⟿ Promote Confidence and Strength (in Men)

carnation (MA)
heliotrope (mi)
bergamot! (mi)
cinnamon! (T)
elderberry (T)

Recommended application: Direct or indirect inhalation

⟿ Promote Self-Confidence (in Women)

carnation (MA)
amber (mi)
elderberry (mi)

Recommended application: Direct or indirect inhalation

⟿ Overcome Aggression

bergamot! (MA)
lavender (mi)
ylang ylang (mi)

>**Recommended application:** Direct or indirect inhalation, bath

⟿ Awaken Pleasant Memories

vanilla (MA)
spearmint (mi)

>**Recommended application:** Bath, direct or indirect inhalation

⟿ Stir Past Life or Genetic Memory

sandalwood (MA)
frankincense! (mi)
myrrh! (mi)
jasmine (mi)
cypress (mi)
mimosa (mi)
hyacinth (mi)
cinnamon! (T)

>**Recommended application:** Bath, direct or indirect inhalation (If using an indirect method, use generously.)

CHAPTER 12

Magickal Blends

Like the previous section on therapeutic blends, this first sampling of magickal fragrances will include exact amounts. However, it cannot be over-emphasized that individual artistry, inspiration, experimentation, and investigation is strongly encouraged. Precise formulae are included only so that it is more clearly seen how a magickal blend is composed. These are but a few of the many possible combinations of oil blends directed to specific magickal purposes. The limits of the field of magickal aromatherapy are governed only by the boundaries of knowledge and instinct of the individual artisan.

Many magicians who entertain requests for aid from the general public will tell you that there are three main areas of need that arise again and again. The root of people's dissatisfaction, when their lives take a bad turn, may often be attributed to a need for protection, love, or money. We would not be complete in addressing magickal working with essential oils if we did not include the blended solutions to these universal ills. Therefore, a few of the possible oil combinations are included for the magickal approach to these types of problems, as well as a few others.

These are but a small sampling of the limitless number of possible blends in magickal aromatherapy, and but a small selection of the many different magickal intentions that may be addressed through the craft of fragrance magick. Using these blends as a base, adventurous (yet responsible) research and experimentation is encouraged. The goal is to develop the most highly effective, best-suited fragrance for a particular magickal purpose. The use of natural inspiration can only enhance the gifts of the art of aromatherapy. After all, the arcane arts and sciences are the tools of the magician. The real magick dwells within the heart and soul of the sorcerer of scents.

Note: Please be aware of oils marked as potential irritants (!).

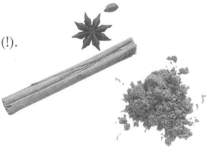

Love

¼ dram gardenia	½ dram rose
¼ dram magnolia	¼ dram jasmine
¼ dram hyacinth	⅛ dram carnation
¼ dram lavender	⅛ dram apple
½ dram musk	½ dram musk
¼ dram ambergris	⅜ dram ambergris
¼ dram vanilla	⅛ dram patchouli

Background and use: May be used as candle dressing, perfume oil, or in a bath.

Universal Unconditional Love

½ dram strawberry	¾ dram ylang ylang
¼ dram apple	¼ dram violet
¼ dram orange!	2 drops cinnamon!

Background and use: These are fairly new blends. It is the New Age mentality that has given strength to the concept of unconditional love. Use as candle dressing, bath, spray, or perfume oil.

Protection

½ dram vetivert	¼ dram juniper
¼ dram galangal	¼ dram pine
¼ dram bay	¼ dram lime
3 drops clove!	¼ dram galangal

Background and use: While these are rooted chiefly in European and Jamaican magick, their usage is universal. Use as candle dressing, spray, bath, floor wash, or personal oil.

Money

½ dram honeysuckle	¼ dram patchouli
¼ dram vanilla	¼ dram heliotrope
¼ dram oakmoss!	¼ dram vanilla
4 drops cinnamon!	¼ dram jasmine

Background and use: These influences are a combination of different cultural influences. They may be equally at home in Mexico, Europe, and the Caribbean. Use as candle dressing, bath, or personal perfume oil.

Psychic Development

½	dram violet	½	dram ylang ylang
¼	dram bay	½	dram mimosa
¼	dram bergamot!	1	drop elderberry

Background and use: Newer New Age creations, use these in candle dressing, oil diffuser, burner, light ring, personal anointing oil, or bath.

Happiness

½	dram apple	½	dram bergamot!
¼	dram orange!	¼	dram gardenia
¼	dram bergamot!	¼	dram ylang ylang
5	drops lemon verbena!	4	drops lavender

Background and use: Bath, spray, floor wash, direct or indirect inhalant.

Health

½	dram cypress	½	dram sandalwood
¼	dram pine	¼	dram myrrh!
¼	dram lily	¼	dram bay
2	drops eucalyptus	3	drops clove!

Background and use: Bath, direct or indirect inhalation.

Spirituality

¼	dram frankincense!	¼	dram cedar
¼	dram myrrh!	¼	dram jasmine
¼	dram sandalwood	¼	dram lotus
¼	dram lemon!	¼	dram rose

Background and use: Inhalant (especially as incense).

Advanced Magickal Blends

Due to the varied nature of the magickal blends in both origin and method of application, each of the magickal formulas includes a short statement indicating the nature, origin, or history of the blend as well as an indication of the possible use of the blended fragrance. Like the presentation of therapeutic remedies, the possible combinations of magickal mixtures is without limit. It would be impossible to include all the potential variances of combinations. Even the inclusion of all those blends that have become a part of my own limited practice would produce an unwieldy formulary. However, with those that have been included, there is a good cross-section of varying blends that are addressed to specific purposes.

The blends included here are of three main types. While the same codes (MA, mi, and T) have been carried over as a guideline for determining the amount of each individual component, there have been some additional codes included specifically for the magickal blends. These will indicate whether the formula is a traditional formula (t), a personal design (g), or a variation adapted from a traditional oil blend (v).

Again, it should be emphasized that, as was the case with the therapeutic blends, the formulae that have been included are written in a loose, non-stringent manner in order to accommodate the individual creativity and expertise of the magickal practitioner.

The system used to catalog these formulae is the creation of different sections for each of the general magickal intentions. These are separated as formulae of Love and Lust, Success and Prosperity, Health, Magickal Empowerment, Ritual Blends, and A Step on the Dark Side. A name cross-reference is included in the appendix. Some of the traditional formulae are known by different names in different cultures but have the same magickal intention.

Love and Lust

⌒ *All Night Long (v)*

jasmine (MA)
vanilla (mi)
musk (mi)

> **Background and use:** Said to eliminate sexual inhibition while increasing stamina. Used to scent the bed chamber in incense or potpourri, or as a personal anointing oil.

⌒ *Alsacian Sex—Female (g)*

musk (MA)
civet (MA)
ambergris (mi)
patchouli (T)

> **Background and use:** Created for women to sexually attract men. Worn as a personal oil.

⌒ *Alsacian Sex—Male (g)*

musk (MA)
ambergris (mi)
muguet (T)

> **Background and use:** This is a variation of an oil originally prepared as a personal oil for the author. Worn by men to sexually arouse and attract women, it was the predecessor to its above female counterpart.

⌒ *Attraction (v)*

patchouli (MA)
lavender (MA)
cedarwood (mi)

> **Background and use:** May be used in sprinkling powder, incense, or oil form. Reported to draw only good things—luck, money, love, success. Some say that this scent should always be worn as a personal oil when looking for a mate.

⟶ *Cleopatra (v)*

heliotrope (MA)
cedarwood (MA)
rose (MA)
frankincense! (T)

> **Background and use:** An especially favored scent of voodoo
> practitioners, Cleopatra may be used in a love spell to anoint a
> pink candle, worn to strengthen and enhance the relationship
> between lovers, or worn to attract a secretly desired stranger.

⟶ *Come and See Me (g)*

patchouli (MA)
clove! (T)

> **Background and use:** Used as a candle anointing oil to
> encourage a loved one to come around for a visit.

⟶ *Come to Me (t)*

rose (MA)
jasmine (mi)
gardenia (mi)
lemon! (T)

> **Background and use:** Often worn near the
> heart (whether by anointing the self or a
> specially prepared ounga bag, a specially
> prepared magickal bag used as a talisman
> for a variety of purposes) to draw a lover.
> This is considered an especially
> potent formula.

Eyes for Me (g)

musk (MA)
civet (MA)
gardenia (MA)
ambergris (mi)
myrrh! (mi)

> **Background and use:** This blend was created in response to a special request for use as a personal or candle anointing oil to stimulate fidelity in a lover.

Follow Me Boy (t)

jasmine (MA)
rose (mi)
vanilla (T)

> **Background and use:** The traditional version of this product, in addition to the pure scents, contained a piece of coral and some gold dust or gold glitter. It was favored by New Orleans prostitutes to ensure that they would make plenty of money through the appreciation of their passions.

Follow Me Girl (g)

myrrh! (MA)
patchouli (MA)
vetivert (mi)
lemon! (mi)
vanilla (mi)
sandalwood (mi)

> **Background and use:** Based on the traditional New Orleans formula, this is an attraction oil created for use by men.

I Tame My Straying Animal (t)

peppermint! (MA)
clove! (mi)
onion oil! (T)

> **Background and use:** This preparation, which originates from Mexico, is intended for use in keeping a wandering lover at home.

Love Oil (v)

gardenia (MA)
jasmine (MA)
sandalwood (MA)
musk (mi)
muguet (mi)

> **Background and use:** While this traditional blend was designed for use in the preparation of incense (often molded in the shape of hearts), the variant blend may also be used as a bath to attract lovers to the user.

Lover Come Back (g)

patchouli (MA)
myrrh! (mi)
clove! (T)

> **Background and use:** By special request, this oil was created to bring back a wandering lover.

La Flamme Oil (v)

musk (MA)
ambergris (mi)
bay (T)
mimosa (T)

> **Background and use:** Used as an anointing oil for candles or talismans, this blend is reported to fix thoughts of you firmly in your lover's mind. It may be used to enhance a lover's sense of excitement toward the user or to bring home a lover that has strayed.

Magnetic Blade (g)

musk (MA)
patchouli (MA)
ambergris (MA)
civet (MA)
cinnamon! (T)

> **Background and use:** This blend was designed by special request for use in love attraction by homosexual men.

Marriage Oil (v)

rose (MA)
pine (MA)
myrrh! (MA)
muguet (MA)

> **Background and use:** Based on a traditional blend, this scent
> was intended to help an unsure suitor gain the confidence to pro-
> pose. It can also be used to scent the home to keep a
> marriage peaceful and happy.

New Orleans' Desire (v)

magnolia (MA)
carnation (MA)
rose (MA)
orange! (MA)
civet (T)
vanilla (T)

> **Background and use:** Based on a blend originally used by ladies
> of the night in nineteenth-century New Orleans, this blend is a
> design for sexual attraction. It is said that its original users
> employed it to not only ensure financial gain for the night but
> also so their clients would return with their friends. The newly
> created version has been used to increase financial gain for those
> in businesses with sexual undertones to increase their incomes
> (i.e., club waitresses, exotic dancers, entertainers, et cetera).

Special Attraction (g)

musk (MA)
heliotrope (mi)
carnation (mi)
ambergris (mi)
cinnamon! (T)

> **Background and use:** By special request, Special Attraction was
> developed for a man who wished to attract women. Reportedly
> very successful, it was worn as a personal oil.

Special Oil #20 (t)

gardenia (MA)
jasmine (MA)
lily of the valley (MA)
sandalwood (MA)

> **Background and use:** A traditional voodoo blend, this oil may be
> used as a general love attraction oil. In conjunction with some
> old voodoo charms, however, it can be used specifically to
> encourage oral sexual activity. These enlist the aid of the voodoo
> loa Aida Hwedo.

Stay at Home (v)

patchouli (MA)
lavender (MA)
cedarwood (MA)
pine (MA)
camphor! (T)

> **Background and use:** Encourages a lover to stay at home by empha-
> sizing the qualities of comfort and stability as well as arousing
> feelings of loyalty and passion to the lover or spouse.

True Love Oil (t)

lily of the valley (MA)
rose (mi)
patchouli (mi)
cinnamon! (T)

> **Background and use:** Used as a
> personal oil to attract and
> bind lasting love.

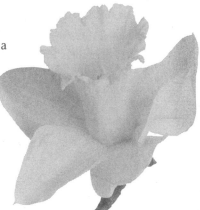

Success and Prosperity

⌐ Better Business (t)

heliotrope (MA)
patchouli (mi)
lavender (mi)

> **Background and use:** May be used as incense or for anointing candles or talismans.

⌐ Bingo (v)

jasmine (MA)
lily of the valley (MA)
bay (mi)
clove! (T)

> **Background and use:** A drop placed in the left shoe or on the bingo markers is used to persuade fortune to smile on the bingo parlor regular.

⌐ Binding Job Oil (g)

heliotrope (MA)
musk (MA)
patchouli (MA)
ambergris (mi)
civet (mi)

> **Background and use:** Specially developed for bringing final resolution to job hunting efforts. Used on an employment application or résumé, this blend is intended to secure an interview. Worn as a personal oil for the interview, it may result in an offer of employment.

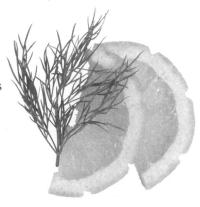

⟋ *Business Attraction (g)*

heliotrope (MΛ)
patchouli (mi)
orange! (mi)
cinnamon! (T)
elderberry (T)

> **Background and use:** Use as an anointing oil on green, pink, and orange candles, or for the preparation of an incense. This blend is especially intended for retail establishments. It is designed to increase sales by establishing a more pleasant, friendly atmosphere in the place of business—making it a place where people want to be and want to spend their money.

⟋ *Crowning Glory Job Oil (v)*

jasmine (MA)
honeysuckle (MA)
amber (MA)
orange! (MA)
gold glitter (pinch)

> **Background and use:** Used for personal or candle anointing for help in the job searching process.

⟋ *Customer Attraction (g)*

rose (MA)
patchouli (MA)
cedarwood (MA)
orange! (MA)
elderberry (T)

> **Background and use:** Used both to bring in customers and to stabilize business. Anoint green candles and burn in the place of business, or make an incense, spray mist, or floor wash from the scent.

Fast Luck (t)

patchouli (MA)
carnation (mi)
mimosa (mi)

> **Background and use:** A blend that seems to span many magickal traditions and cultures, this oil is designed to bring in money quickly. It may be used as a personal oil, to anoint green or gold candles, or as an anointing for talismans.

Gambler's Oil (t)

lily of the valley (MA)
rose (MA)
sandalwood (MA)
mimosa (MA)
cinnamon! (T)

> **Background and use:** The gambler's good luck in a bottle. A traditional scent used to enhance the gifts of Lady Luck.

Good Luck (v)

patchouli (MA)
vetivert (MA)
jasmine (MA)
lemon! (mi)
rose (mi)

> **Background and use:** Simply worn as a personal oil or in a bath to encourage good things to be drawn to the user.

Job Oil (t)

heliotrope (MA)
hyacinth (MA)
patchouli (mi)
cinnamon! (T)

> **Background and use:** A personal anointing or ritual anointing oil used to speed up the job searching process and ensure its success.

Lottery (g)

patchouli (MA)
rose (mi)
lemon! (mi)

Background and use: An often requested blend to help gain an edge in the lottery drawings. Anoint the corners of the ticket with the oil.

Money Drawing (t)

patchouli (MA)
pine (mi)
bay (mi)

Background and use: Another magickal blend common to many different magickal practices, it is used for personal or ritual anointing to draw money to the user.

Prosperity (g)

gardenia (MA)
patchouli (mi)
cinnamon! (T)

Background and use: A special design, this oil has been reported to be especially effective when a few drops are used to anoint the checkbook.

Road Opener (t)

jasmine (MA)
bay (mi)
hyacinth (mi)
cinnamon! (T)

Background and use: Originally a Mexican blend, this mixture is often used in conjunction with other oils to open the door to new opportunities or to clear the road of any obstacles.

Sales (g)

heliotrope (MA)
jasmine (MA)
gardenia (mi)
magnolia (mi)
apple (mi)
mimosa (mi)
vanilla (T)
orange! (T)

> **Background and use:** Designed to enhance the natural sales skill of the career salesperson when used as a personal oil.

School Oil (g)

sandalwood (MA)
lavender (mi)
pine (mi)
musk (mi)
cinnamon! (T)

> **Background and use:** Used to enhance academic skills for the student. Anointing is done at the forehead, wrists, and temples.

Sesame Customer Attraction (v)

rose (MA)
patchouli (MA)
cedarwood (MA)
orange! (MA)

> **Background and use:** The original formula for this blend was created for casting out evil influence. However, when used in the production of incense, this modified formula may be used to draw in customers to a business.

Success (t)

heliotrope (MA)
patchouli (mi)
lavender (mi)

> **Background and use:** Common to many magickal traditions, this oil is used in ritual and/or candle anointing to encourage general success in all undertakings.

Test Pass (g)

rose (MA)
lily of the valley (MA)
lavender (mi)
violet (mi)

> **Background and use:** This oil was created by special request. The person for whom it was originally produced won high honors in a nationwide academic competition and a college scholarship.

Protection and Well-Being

Cleansing (t)

lotus (MA)
frankincense! (MA)
amber (MA)
cedarwood (MA)

> **Background and use:** This is a general purpose purifying blend. Used in incense or water, it is intended to cleanse the premises of any negative or unwanted energies.

Court Case (t)

hyacinth (MA)
lily of the valley (mi)
lavender (mi)

> **Background and use:** A favored oil for those who find themselves on the wrong side of the legal process. This blend is designed to protect the user against the wrath of the court and to obtain a judgment that is favorable. Most often this blend is used as an anointing oil for candles or for the person.

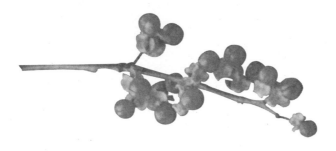

⁓ *Doublecross (v)*

myrrh! (MA)
mimosa (MA)
jasmine (MA)
patchouli (MA)
clove! (T)

> **Background and use:** A magickal blend that spans the disciplines of different traditions in folk magic, Doublecross was created to turn back any negative magic or undo the hex of an adversary practitioner.

⁓ *Dragon's Blood (v)*

jasmine (MA)
cedarwood (mi)
cyclamen (mi)
cinnamon! (T)
wintergreen! (T)
dragon's blood (the plant resin—a pinch)

> **Background and use:** Favored especially by Mexican practitioners, this oil has been employed as protective blend for use in anointing candles and talismans and for making protective incense.

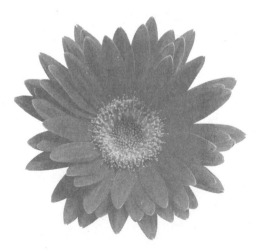

~⁀ *Happy Home (t)*

rose (MA)
gardenia (MA)
myrrh! (MA)
mimosa (MA)
eucalyptus (T)

> **Background and use:** May be used in waters, spray mists, incense, or as a candle dressing to maintain or restore peace and serenity in the home.

~⁀ *Jinx Removing (t)*

rose (MA)
clove! (mi)
wintergreen! (mi)
cinnamon! (T)

> **Background and use:** A blend found throughout different cultures and magickal traditions, this preparation is used on candles and in incense to undo a curse.

~⁀ *Just Judge (t)*

patchouli (MA)
sandalwood (MA)
hyacinth (mi)
dragon's blood (pinch)

> **Background and use:** Another preparation to protect against negative results in court cases, Just Judge is said to guarantee favor, compassion, and fairness from the magistrate's bench.

~⁀ *Needed Changes (v)*

sandalwood (MA)
mimosa (mi)
hyacinth (mi)
cinnamon! (T)

> **Background and use:** Worn as a personal oil or as an anointing oil for candles or in incense, this oil was created to promote changes for the better in one's life.

⌒⌒ *Pentatruck (t)*

myrrh! (MA)
bay (mi)
cinnamon! (T)
clove! (T)

> **Background and use:** Specifically designed as a protection blend for use as an anointing oil with the seal of Solomon.

⌒⌒ *Protection (g)*

frankincense! (MA)
myrrh! (MA)
cedarwood (mi)

> **Background and use:** This blend was specially requested for dealing with magickal workings of some specific traditions. It is reported to be effective specifically in protecting against the workings of Egyptian and Sumerian magick.

⌒⌒ *General Protection (g)*

frankincense! (MA)
sandalwood (MA)
amber (mi)

> **Background and use:** This blend may be used in accordance with any specific magickal rite, spell, or practice related to protection. It was designed as a general purpose blend to accommodate a wide array of needs.

⌒⌒ *Reversing (t)*

lemon! (MA)
rosemary! (mi)
spikenard (mi)
rose (mi)
peppermint! (T)

> **Background and use:** Specifically intended as a reply to magickal attack, this blended oil not only is intended to protect against the attack but to return its impact to the sender.

Salvation Oil (t)

rose (MA)
camphor! (T)

> **Background and use:** Originating from Mexico, this blend is used
> to relieve the user of negative influences surrounding him or her
> by enveloping them in a sphere of holy blessings.

Sealing Oil (v)

lemon verbena! (MA)
amber (mi)
vetivert (mi)
lavender (mi)
galangal (mi)

> **Background and use:** Following the remedy of the effects of illness
> or magickal attack, this preparation is used in a bath or as an
> anointing oil to seal the goodness in and the undesirable out.
> It can be used to prevent a recurrence of the conditions that
> needed to be relieved in the first place.

St. Michael (v)

frankincense! (MA)
sandalwood (mi)
carnation (mi)
cinnamon! (T)
clove! (T)

> **Background and use:** Sometimes
> known as "Fiery Wall of
> Protection Oil," this blend is
> specially designed to enlist the
> aid of St. Michael for protection.
> It may be made into a bath, used
> in candle spells, as an anointing
> oil to consecrate a St. Michael's
> medal for protection, or worn as a
> personal oil. If used as a personal oil, it
> may need to be diluted into a carrier oil.
> Some of the ingredients will act as certain
> irritants to sensitive skin.

St. Michael for Children (g)

carnation (MA)
frankincense! (mi)
sandalwood (mi)
lavender (T)

> **Background and use:** A gentler version of the traditional oil designed for use with children. Because the irritant elements have been omitted, it is less likely to cause problems with children's soft, sensitive skin tissues.

Tetragrammaton (t)

frankincense! (MA)
cedarwood (MA)
mimosa (mi)
lemon! (mi)

> **Background and use:** Especially intended for protection in conjunction with the ancient talisman of the same name.

Uncrossing (t)

rose (MA)
carnation (mi)
bay (T)
clove! (T)

> **Background and use:** A traditional blend intended to undo negative influences, to cleanse and protect.

Health

It should be noted that while there are many available therapeutic oils for treating various ailments, this can also be approached from a magickal perspective. It is also important to note that those preparations included in the therapeutic formulary are not without merit to those who prefer to deal with illness magickally. Through the use of sympathetic magick, the healing virtues of the therapeutic blends may be transferred to an individual through an outside medium, such as a candle or fith-fath (or so-called "voodoo doll"). Therefore, in undertaking the task of remedying an ailment through magickal healing rites, it is strongly suggested that the therapeutic blends be considered for magickal use as well as the applications for which they were originally designed.

In addition, there are many practitioners who combine the benefits of therapeutic aromatherapy with magickal practices. Although one may perform a traditional magickal rite of healing, the use of therapeutic massage or aromatherapy healing may be combined with that rite. It is a wise worker of the healing magicks that takes advantage of all the possible benefits laid at his or her disposal.

Anger Fade (g)

rose (MA)
amber (MA)
gardenia (mi)
carnation (mi)
camphor! (T)

> **Background and use:** This blend, although originally designed as a magickal preparation, has since been proven a suitable preparation for therapeutic use through inhalation therapy. As a magickal blend, however, it was designed to be used as a single drop anointing application on the forehead (over the third eye).

Calming Oil (g)

rose (MA)
amber (MA)
gardenia (mi)
eucalyptus (T)

> **Background and use:** This blend also may be used both magickally and therapeutically in very much the same manner as Anger Fade, its predecessor. The major difference between the two preparations is that Anger Fade was developed to bring instantaneous results while Calming Oil is broader-based, intended for ongoing relief of stressful conditions.

⟿ *Cleansing Oil (v)*

lotus (MA)
frankincense! (MA)
amber (MA)
cedarwood (MA)

> **Background and use:** Most traditions in magickal practice have a cleansing or purifying blend in their arsenals. While these are often used for ritual cleansing, they may also be employed for the relief of non-specific ailments. They are not recommended so much for distinct illnesses but for a case of the blahs. A cleansing bath may be responsible for a major turnaround.

⟿ *Hangover Oil (g)*

juniper (MA)
rosemary! (mi)
lavender (mi)
orange! (mi)

> **Background and use:** A specifically requested blend, this preparation was designed to be used when the festivities of the night before spill into the morning after. It should be especially effective in use as a bath treatment.

⟿ *Healing (t)*

cedarwood (MA)
carnation (MA)
pine (MA)
cypress (MA)

> **Background and use:** A general application blend, this magickal preparation may be used as an all-purpose healer in conjunction with any desired transmittal method—as an anointing oil for candles or talismans, a bath, or a personal oil.

Health Oil (t)

gardenia (MA)
carnation (mi)
rose (mi)
citronella! (T)

> **Background and use:** Especially recommended for baths and candle magick.

No Drink (g)

juniper (MA)
myrrh! (MA)
lavender (mi)
rose (mi)
ylang ylang (mi)
rosemary! (mi)

> **Background and use:** Often used in combination with a spiritual oil, confidence building oil, or a universal love type of blend, this scent was created to help those who are either prone to alcoholism or who just experience negative effects in their lives due to excessive alcohol consumption. Its purpose is to help the individual to break free from a physical or mental dependency on the stimulus.

Rising Sun (g)

carnation (MA)
heliotrope (mi)
bergamot! (mi)
cinnamon! (T)
elderberry (T)

> **Background and use:** Rising Sun was designed in response to an apparent need in the community. It is intended to bolster inner strength in men. As such, it is a confidence builder and a spiritual, mental, and physical strengthener—it brings out the highest virtues of manhood, including strength and honor. It acts almost as a tonic in revitalizing the spiritual and physical well-being.

⁓ *Sun Glow Health Oil (g)*

jasmine (MA)
honeysuckle (MA)
amber (MA)
orange! (MA)
elderberry (T)

Background and use: The origin of this particular oil was rooted in error. While preparing a totally different blend, some ingredients were mistakenly included in the mix. The resulting formula turned out to be a successful healing tool.

This was initially used as a chakra anointing oil to effect the process of restoring health. The woman who first used Sun Glow Health Oil was very happy with the results. Having a chronic condition that forced her to use a walker in order to have any mobility, after treating her chakra points with the remedy she was able to walk with only the use of a cane. Sometimes she could even do without this aid. The effects of the application offered her relief for several hours at a time.

⁓ *Sun Glow Health Oil II (g)*

hyacinth (MA)
elderberry (MA)
amber (MA)
orange! (MA)

Background and use: The request from this design originated from the same woman who first benefited from the use of Sun Glow Health Oil. After using the blend for several weeks and enjoying the benefits, she issued a challenge to produce a healing blend that was stronger and more enduring. The resulting blend brought her daily uses down to one or two per day instead of one every three to five hours.

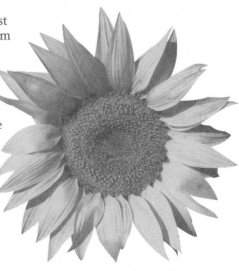

Waxing Moon (g)

carnation (MA)
amber (MA)
elderberry (MA)

> **Background and use:** This is the female counterpart to Rising Sun. Often used as a personal anointing oil, it is intended to bring out the inner strength and beauty in women. With the fulfillment of womanhood virtues also comes increased energies and robust health.

Magickal Empowerment

Astral Travel (g)

frankincense! (MA)
myrrh! (MA)
cypress (MA)
jasmine (MA)

> **Background and use:** The design of this oil blend was conceived with the intention of helping those encountering difficulty in successfully exploring astral travel. It has reportedly not only been an asset to the new voyager to astral worlds but has also helped the more experienced astral traveler to gain access to the unseen planes. It may be used as an incense but is more preferred as a personal anointing oil.

Celtic Virtue (g)

bay (MA)
bergamot! (MA)
juniper (MA)
pine (mi)
carnation (mi)
apple (T)
elderberry (T)

> **Background and use:** By special request, Celtic Virtue was designed to bring out the old Celtic values of honor, courage, strength, justice, and camaraderie. It is used as an anointing oil and helps to awaken genetic, or ancestral, memories for those who are following a spiritual path reflecting the old Celtic cultures.

Concentration (v)

myrrh! (MA)
violet (mi)
cinnamon! (T)

> **Background and use:** Used as a personal anointing oil, incense, or chakra treatment, this blend is designed to enhance the mental awareness of the individual, enabling him or her to function at his or her best.

Courage (v)

jasmine (MA)
pine (mi)
bay (T)
clove! (T)

> **Background and use:** An adaptation of a traditional formula, this preparation is intended to bring out and enhance an individual's innate qualities of courage and conviction.

Divination (v)

musk (MA)
ambergris (mi)
vetivert (mi)
violet (mi)
lilac (mi)

> **Background and use:** Divination oil is intended to open up the psychic facilities for clarity and increased insight. It is often used as an anointing oil on the forehead (third eye) and the temples.

Divine Man (v)

patchouli (MA)
pine (mi)
cedarwood (mi)

> **Background and use:** A variation of a formula known by some as God Oil, the purpose of this blend is to bring out a man's spirituality, aligning his mind, heart, and soul with the spirit of the gods who have been worshipped throughout the history of the world's religions.

⌇ *Divine Woman (v)*

frankincense! (MA)
sandalwood (MA)
jasmine (MA)
lotus (MA)
elderberry (T)

> **Background and use:** A variation of a formula known by some as
> Goddess Oil, the purpose of this blend is to bring out a woman's
> spirituality, aligning her mind, heart, and soul with the spirit of
> the goddesses who have been worshiped throughout the history
> of the world's religions.

⌇ *Dreams (g)*

magnolia (MA)
mimosa (MA)
orange! (MA)
violet (MA)

> **Background and use:** This blend is intended to enhance the quality
> of dreams and provide knowledge and psychic insights to the
> dreamer who uses it. It may be used as a personal anointing oil,
> as an anointing for external agents in sympathetic magick, or
> used in any of the methods of application designed to scent
> the room in which the individual sleeps.

⌇ *Fantasy (g)*

sandalwood (MA)
musk (mi)
galangal (mi)
cinnamon! (T)
clove! (T)

> **Background and use:** Fantasy Oil originated with the spirit of the
> New Age. It was created to enhance the imagination and the
> sense of fantasy. Many of the traditional arts and sciences, like
> divination, healing, and visualization, are rooted
> in the foundation of fertile imagination.
> To develop skill in these endeavors it may
> be necessary to first develop a sound
> sense of free-flowing fantasy.

Meditation (g)

gardenia (MA)
violet (MA)
mimosa (MA)
myrrh! (MA)

> **Background and use:** Used as an anointing oil on the crown and
> head chakras, meditation oil can enhance the depth of meditative
> journeys. It may also enhance the quality of insightful realization
> and any other benefits of meditation techniques.

Psychic Power (g)

cedarwood (MA)
myrrh! (MA)
violet (MA)
musk (mi)
ambergris (mi)

> **Background and use:** This is a preparation that is designed to do
> for the development of psychic facilities what Power Oil does
> for magickal skills.

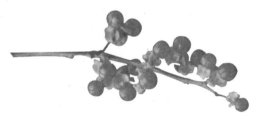

Spiritual Oil (t)

sandalwood (MA)
frankincense! (MA)
rose (MA)
cedarwood (mi)
jasmine (mi)

> **Background and use:** As an anointing oil, fragrant bath, or incense, this blend promotes the attainment of higher levels of spiritual realization. It has a dual effect in that it brings to the surface one's own spirituality while also inviting the goodness of external forces to come to the user.

Vision Quest (g)

cedarwood (MA)
hyacinth (mi)
violet (mi)

> **Background and use:** Originally developed for an individual who leads people on a spiritual journey of self-discovery, this preparation may help to open up the individual seeker enough to expedite his or her journey through the world of spiritual insight and attainment. It is intended for use primarily as a personal anointing oil.

Miscellaneous Oils

In addition to addressing specific types of magickal empowerment, it should be noted that the observation of the ancient practices of the old arts may bring an empowerment of their own through personal attainment. Some of these types of empowerment oils may deal with the identification of an individual with the particular criteria of different practices. In astrology, the specific empowerment fragrances may be tied to zodiac signs, planets, or elements. One of the things that should be remembered about the astrological oils is that while there are traditional values accorded to each of the astrological categories, there are also preconceived notions that people have about themselves. Often, one aspect or another of a sign, planet, or element is taken to heart to the exclusion of the others. As a result, though the oil formula may be true to its purpose, it may not be favored by the individual who is aligned with its particular influences. For example, being a Scorpio, it was a natural step for me to want to experiment with the Scorpio oil once it was developed. On first contact, it was not a true reflection of what I considered Scorpio traits to be. Upon further analysis, however, it seems that the oil is uniquely suited to Scorpio influence. The problem was that there were some aspects of the Scorpio personality that were more highly valued, personally, than others. Thoughts of adjusting the formula were discarded. The end result was that it became possible, armed with a more accurate blend, to more fully develop and appreciate the less dramatic yet more healthily stabilizing virtues of the Scorpio personality.

Likewise, in speaking with many different people native to different signs of the zodiac, there are many who carry a slanted view of their own signs. However, remaining true to the preparation of a truly reflective blend of the specific influences, one can more clearly see the virtues that are innately available and overcome any weaknesses that may be inherent in the force of their particular zodiac sign. Using the true fragrances for astrological influences can be not only enlightening but also a balancing, stabilizing, clarifying experience.

Another area of empowerment may be seen through chakra work. There are individual oils for each of the traditional chakra gates. These may be used for healing, insight, spiritual cleansing, and empowerment.

The Astrology Oils (g)

Zodiac Signs (g)

⟳ Aquarius

jasmine (MA)
lavender (mi)
patchouli (mi)
lemon! (T)

⟳ Aries

rose (MA)
pine (mi)
lemon! (mi)
cinnamon! (T)

⟳ Cancer

lily of the valley (MA)
gardenia (mi)
jasmine (mi)
camphor! (T)
clove! (T)

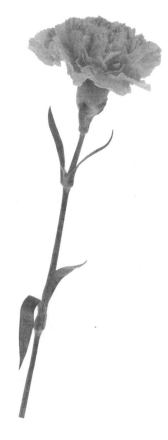

⟳ Capricorn

carnation (MA)
pine (mi)

⟳ Gemini

violet (MA)
lavender (MA)
heliotrope (MA)
mimosa (MA)
frankincense! (MA)

Leo

rose (MA)
patchouli (MA)
musk (mi)
lemon! (mi)

Pisces

lavender (MA)
carnation (MA)
lilac (MA)
patchouli (MA)

Scorpio

myrrh! (MA)
hyacinth (MA)
pine (MA)
lemon! (MA)
cinnamon! (T)

Virgo

rose (MA)
lavender (MA)
patchouli (MA)
honeysuckle (mi)
wintergreen! (mi)
mimosa (mi)
bay (T)

Libra

lily of the valley (MA)
lavender (mi)
lemon! (T)

Sagittarius

pine (MA)
musk (MA)
muguet (MA)
myrrh! (mi)
hyacinth (mi)

Taurus

ambergris (MA)
patchouli (MA)
musk (MA)
jasmine (MA)
bay (T)

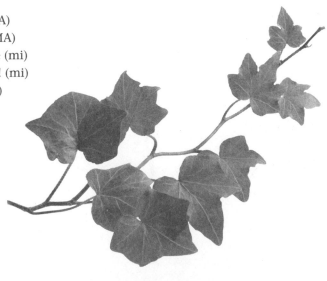

Planets (g)

Jupiter

frankincense! (MA)
cedarwood (MA)
hyacinth (mi)
clove! (T)

Mars

pine (MA)
frankincense! (MA)
carnation (mi)
clove! (T)
dragon's blood (pinch)

Mercury

muguet (MA)
lily of the valley (mi)
lavender (mi)
violet (mi)
eucalyptus (T)

Moon

lily of the valley (MA)
sandalwood (mi)
jasmine (mi)
camphor! (T)

Neptune

mimosa (MA)
rose (MA)
ambergris (mi)

Pluto

musk (MA)
frankincense! (mi)
hyacinth (mi)

Saturn

myrrh! (MA)
patchouli (MA)
lotus (mi)
elderberry (T)

Sun

frankincense! (MA)
heliotrope (mi)
bay (mi)
carnation (mi)
cinnamon! (T)

Uranus

musk (MA)
sandalwood (MA)
rose (mi)

Venus

jasmine (MA)
rose (mi)
ambergris (mi)
muguet (mi)
lavender (mi)
cinnamon! (T)

Elements (g)

⌒ Air

lavender (MA)
lily of the valley (MA)
lilac (mi)

⌒ Earth

pine (MA)
cypress (MA)
patchouli (MA)
oakmoss! (mi)

⌒ Fire

frankincense! (MA)
sandalwood (mi)
carnation (mi)
cinnamon! (T)
clove! (T)

⌒ Water

mimosa (MA)
lotus (MA)
sandalwood (MA)
rose (mi)
cucumber (mi)

The Chakra Oils (g)

⌒ Balancing Oil

lemon! (MA)
orange! (MA)
lavender (MA)
myrrh! (MA)
clove! (T)

⌒ Base Chakra

musk (MA)
ambergris (mi)
civet (mi)
muguet (mi)
cinnamon! (T)

⌒ Belly Chakra

frankincense! (MA)
lemon verbena! (MA)
honeysuckle (mi)
galangal (mi)

⌒ Crown Chakra

myrrh! (MA)
lotus (mi)
frankincense! (mi)
camphor! (T)

Head Chakra

carnation (MA)
lavender (MA)
rosemary! (mi)
spikenard (mi)

Heart Chakra

cedarwood (MA)
mimosa (MA)
rosemary! (mi)
clove! (T)

Spine Chakra

orange! (MA)
oakmoss! (mi)
sandalwood (mi)

Throat Chakra

vanilla (MA)
violet (mi)
ylang ylang (mi)
eucalyptus (T)

Ritual Blends

Abramelin (t)

myrrh! (MA)
galangal (MA)
cinnamon! (T)

Background and use: This is a special blend designed for use with ritual work in accordance with the writings of the old magician as preserved in the writings *Abramelin the Mage*.

Altar Oil (t)

frankincense! (MA)
myrrh! (MA)
rose (MA)
sandalwood (MA)

Background and use: An almost universally usable blend, it is used to sanctify the ritual space and the sacred altar, and as a candle anointing oil.

Blessing Oil (v)

myrrh! (MA)
frankincense! (MA)
cedarwood (MA)
lemon verbena! (MA)

> **Background and use:** Many different traditions of magick use an all-purpose fragrance for ritual work. This particular blend could be employed in a variety of different magickal traditions as a personal or sacred ritual implement anointing oil or made into a bath or incense.

Celtic Spirit (g)

sandalwood (MA)
cypress (MA)
juniper (MA)
elderberry (mi)
apple (mi)

> **Background and use:** Requested specifically by a modern-day Celtic clan, this blend was designed for use in Celtic tradition ritual work. It is intended to arouse the spirit of the old Celts in religious and magickal rites and is most frequently used as a personal anointing oil.

Druidic Holy Oil (v)

cedarwood (MA)
frankincense! (mi)
sandalwood (mi)
heliotrope (mi)
cinnamon! (T)

> **Background and use:** Inspired by Druidic magick, this scent was designed for use specifically in the ritual work of the old Druids. It is well suited for use as an anointing oil or in incense.

Dryad (g)

musk (MA)
oakmoss! (mi)
civet (T)
vanilla (T)

> **Background and use:** An excellent blend for pursuing the arts
> of natural magick, this preparation was specially designed
> for contacting the elemental spirits of the earth.

Egyptian Temple (t)

myrrh! (MA)
frankincense! (MA)
lotus (MA)
mimosa (mi)
ambergris (mi)

> **Background and use:** This is an exotic blend especially for use as
> an anointing oil or as an incense for practitioners of the Egyptian
> magickal arts.

Enchantment (g)

musk (MA)
rose (mi)
wintergreen! (T)

> **Background and use:** Used as an anointing oil, a bath, or as an
> incense, this fragrance helps to set the mood for works of
> magick by establishing a dreamy, fluid atmosphere.

Golden Dawn (t)

pine (MA)
myrrh! (MA)
cedarwood (mi)
cinnamon! (T)

> **Background and use:** Dedicated to the practitioners of this
> certain devotion of ceremonial magick, this very male scent
> is often employed in ritual work by celebrants of the Order
> of the Golden Dawn.

⌒ *High Altar (t)*

frankincense! (MA)
myrrh! (mi)
cedarwood (mi)
cinnamon! (T)

> **Background and use:** An important oil in many magickal
> disciplines, this blend is used to purify and bless any sacred
> working tools and the sacred space, as well as to anoint and bless.

⌒ *High Altar (v)*

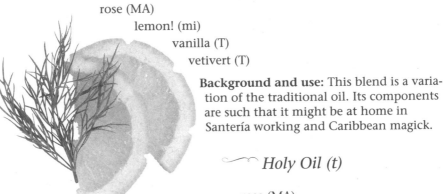

rose (MA)
lemon! (mi)
vanilla (T)
vetivert (T)

> **Background and use:** This blend is a varia-
> tion of the traditional oil. Its components
> are such that it might be at home in
> Santería working and Caribbean magick.

⌒ *Holy Oil (t)*

rose (MA)
lily of the valley (MA)

Background and use: While the elements of this particular blend
are ideally suited for those who follow magick based in a Christian
ideology, the blend may be used as a bath or anointing oil for
almost any discipline. It can also be made into a general purpose
incense.

⌒ *Holy Trinity (t)*

lemon! (MA)
frankincense! (MA)
lily of the valley (mi)

> **Background and use:** Favored by the followers of Santería, this
> blend is well suited for application as an anointing oil or for the
> preparation of a ritual space through use in incense or spray mist.

King Solomon (t)

frankincense! (MA)
myrrh! (MA)
rose (MA)
bay (mi)
jasmine (mi)

> **Background and use:** Although ideal for anointing the seals presented in the Kabbalistic treatise by Solomon, this blend is also favored as a power oil by practitioners of many alternate systems of magick.

Minoan Oil (t)

cedarwood (MA)
patchouli (MA)
oakmoss! (mi)
sandalwood (mi)
musk (mi)
ambergris (mi)
hyacinth (mi)
myrrh! (mi)
rose (mi)

> **Background and use:** This is a blend dedicated for the ritual use of the modern-day counterparts of the adherents of an ancient order of priests.

Moon Oil (v)

lily of the valley (MA)
sandalwood (mi)
jasmine (mi)
camphor! (T)

> **Background and use:** While the original Moon scent was composed of raw herbs that were burned as incense, this variation adds some versatility of use for those who follow the magick of the lunar tides. It is especially favored in rites of fertility.

Obeah (t)

myrrh! (MA)
patchouli (MA)
galangal (MA)
jasmine (mi)
lemon! (mi)

> **Background and use:** Out of Africa and into the hands of the
> well-known Voodoo kings and queens of Louisiana, this oil was
> designed for use in anointing the magick staff, or Obeah stick.
> It has since gained popularity as an all-purpose ritual scent
> and power oil.

Power (v)

patchouli (MA)
jasmine (MA)
gardenia (mi)
camphor! (T)

> **Background and use:** While this blend is intended to enhance
> the magick of the practitioner, it may also be used as a personal
> perfume oil by working practitioners of magick to maintain their
> strength at a maximum level in and out of the ritual space.

Rose of Crucifixion (t)

rose (MA)
clove! (T)
cinnamon! (T)

> **Background and use:** Another holy oil, this blend is especially
> favored by many of the *brujeria*, or practitioners of magick
> in Mexico.

Wicca (g)

patchouli (MA)
violet (MA)
sandalwood (MA)
ambergris (MA)
cinnamon! (T)
camphor! (T)

> **Background and use:** Dedicated to the practitioners of modern-day
> witchcraft, this special blend embraces their magickal workings.

Dedicated to the Gods and Goddesses

There are some scents that are dedicated to the honor of a specific deity. For those followers of the ways of magick who traditionally choose a patron deity, these can be used as a personal scent to align them with their chosen benefactor. Others may utilize a specific scent in a rite honoring a certain god or goddess. Still others employ the different scents to appeal for the aid of a specific deity or to petition that the special virtues of a specific deity be granted.

Aphrodite

gardenia (MA)
rose (MA)
lilac (T)

Apollo

cedarwood (MA)
ambergris (mi)
hyacinth (mi)

Astarte

sandalwood (MA)
rose (MA)
lemon! (MA)
jasmine (MA)

Athena

rose (MA)
gardenia (mi)
sandalwood (T)
myrrh! (T)
frankincense! (T)

Bacchus

jasmine (MA)
sandalwood (MA)
oakmoss (MA)!
pine (MA)

Cerridwen

sandalwood (MA)
rose (MA)
jasmine (mi)
orange! (mi)
patchouli (mi)
civet (mi)
camphor! (T)

Cernunnos

musk (MA)
sandalwood (MA)
frankincense! (MA)
pine (MA)
civet (mi)
cinnamon! (T)

Circe

lotus (MA)
lily of the valley (MA)
musk (MA)
muguet (MA)
clove! (T)
eucalyptus (T)
wintergreen! (T)

Demeter

oakmoss! (MA)
carnation (mi)
pine (T)
jasmine (T)
hyacinth (T)

Diana

jasmine (MA)
sandalwood (mi)
myrrh! (mi)
pine (T)

Hecate

mimosa (MA)
lavender (MA)
camphor! (T)
cedarwood (MA)
lily of the valley (mi)
benzoin (mi)

Hermes

cedarwood (MA)
lily of the valley (mi)
benzoin (mi)

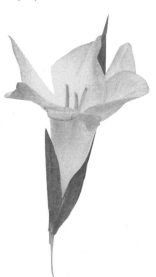

Horus

frankincense! (MA)
myrrh! (MA)
heliotrope (MA)
lotus (mi)
orange! (mi)

Ishtar

sandalwood (MA)
rose (MA)
lemon verbena! (MA)
jasmine (MA)

Isis

myrrh! (MA)
lemon! (MA)
frankincense! (mi)
muguet (mi)
mimosa (mi)
lotus (mi)

Kore

rose (MA)
lavender (MA)
lily of the valley (MA)
bay (mi)
lemon! (mi)

Nefertiti

myrrh! (MA)
lotus! (MA)
gardenia (MA)
lemon! (mi)
muguet (mi)

Woden

oakmoss! (MA)
myrrh! (MA)
sandalwood (MA)
rose (MA)

Kali

mimosa (MA)
lotus (MA)
galangal (MA)
civet (MA)
clove! (T)

Luna

jasmine (MA)
rose (MA)
lotus (mi)
camphor! (T)

Pan

pine (MA)
cedarwood (MA)
patchouli (MA)
ambergris (MA)

Zeus

oakmoss! (MA)
honeysuckle (MA)
sandalwood (MA)
cedarwood (MA)

A Step on the Dark Side

There are multitudes of volumes written on rites of magick, white and black. It should be remembered that it is the intention that lies behind the work that categorizes the type of magick, and not the rite or magickal process itself. Within this book, the emphasis has been placed on the responsibility of the aromatherapist, whether involved in an act of healing or a magickal endeavor. It is without question that the one who blends and uses essential oils is, at the very least, involved in creating change in another's life.

Some may question the virtue of altering another's destiny through the use of natural arts and sciences, and not without some valid foundation. For this reason, personal belief dictates that magick is not truly black or white but different shades of gray. Even when the apparent results of a magickal undertaking are positive, we cannot assume that we had the ethical right to enter into the magickal process in the first place—or, indeed, that the outcome would have been any different had we left it alone.

That being said, there are some undertakings that are obviously of a darker gray than others. When we try to help a fellow spirit, we may well be doing an honorable act—whether or not we may be judged as having the right to do it! However, when we control and manipulate through the ancient arts and when we alter fates to coincide with our own desires or to meet selfish ends, it is more than the virtue of the method that is in question: our own motives are suspect.

Still, it would be an act of neglect to ignore the formulae that are borne of the darker side of magickal practice. The oldest of magickal traditions are not without a few blends directed toward the darker purposes. For this reason, and in order to offer this presentation as a complete sourcebook, the darker blends are included here for reference.

Bend Over Oil (t)

rose (MA)
frankincense! (MA)
honeysuckle (MA)
vetivert (MA)

> **Background and use:** Intended to bend another to the will of the magickal practitioner, this oil is well suited for anointing candles or fith faths (voodoo dolls).

Black Arts (v)

patchouli (MA)
carnation (MA)
pine (mi)
camphor! (T)

> **Background and use:** As there are general purpose blends for
> positive ritual work, such as blessing or altar oil, so the darker side
> has its own general purpose preparations. This one might be used
> as a personal anointing oil or in a bath to temper the mood of the
> practitioner for the ritual work about to be done, as a candle or
> altar anointing oil to set the tone of the ritual space, or in the
> actual magickal act as a directive for the magickal energies raised.

Black Cat (v)

myrrh! (MA)
bay (mi)
sage! (mi)

> **Note:** The original version of this blend also included three black
> cat hairs. As a matter of personal preference and belief, no animal
> parts appear in any of the blends in this formulary.

> **Background and use:** Most often employed as a hexing oil, this oil
> may also be used in rites of luck and love.

Break Up Oil (t)

lavender (MA)
bay (mi)
elderberry (T)
cinnamon! (T)

> **Background and use:** Intended to separate a couple in love, this oil
> is used as an anointing oil for candle working.

Commanding Oil (t)

frankincense! (MA)
myrrh! (MA)
bay (mi)
cinnamon! (T)

> **Background and use:** Used as an anointing oil on candles to bend
> another person to the magician's will.

Confusion (t)

vetivert (MA)
lavender (MA)
galangal (mi)

> **Background and use:** Used in candle magick, waters, or sprinkling
> powders to confuse an enemy.

Controlling Oil (v)

patchouli (MA)
bay (mi)
sandalwood (mi)
pine (mi)
cinnamon! (T)

> **Background and use:** This preparation is yet another blend
> designed to subjugate the will of another to that of the
> magickal practitioner.

Convince (t)

jasmine (MA)
violet (mi)
clove! (T)

> **Background and use:** While this blend must be considered a dark
> side oil because it is designed to manipulate the will of another,
> it should be noted that it is a softer approach to persuasion. It is
> intended to sway another to the magician's way of thinking rather
> than to force the subject to act under the practitioner's will.

Counteracting Oil (v)

lemon verbena! (MA)
rose (MA)
lily of the valley (MA)
bay (mi)
lavender (mi)

> **Background and use:** Used as a candle anointing oil, this blend is
> designed to undo the magick of a fellow practitioner working
> against the magician.

Do As I Say (t)

frankincense! (MA)
myrrh! (MA)
dragon's blood (pinch)

> **Background and use:** One of the few blends that includes
> ingredients from the herbalist's shelf as well as the aromatherapy
> lab, this is another oil intended to control the will of another.
> It is very popular for use in candle magick.

Domination Oil (v)

myrrh! (MA)
bay (mi)
sandalwood (mi)
cinnamon! (T)

> **Background and use:** This blend is used to dominate the will of
> another in magickal working.

Flying Devil (v)

patchouli (MA)
juniper (MA)
vetivert (MA)
myrrh! (mi)
galangal (mi)

> **Background and use:** Used to
> exact revenge on an enemy,
> this mixture is said to enlist
> the aids of demon spirits who
> take pleasure in the payback.

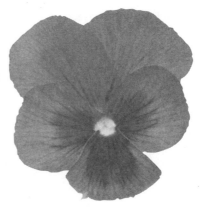

Get Away (v)

bay (MA)
camphor! (T)
eucalyptus (T)
clove! (T)
citronella! (T)

> **Background and use:** In candle magick, waters, and powders, this blend is used to send an enemy or undesirable in the opposite direction.

Hate Oil (v)

galangal (MA)
pine (MA)
camphor! (T)
clove! (T)

> **Background and use:** Used in hexing rituals, this blended oil is intended to wreak havoc on the life of an enemy.

Jury Winning Oil (t)

hyacinth (MA)
lily of the valley (MA)
lavender (mi)

> **Background and use:** This blend, while not truly of a malevolent nature, is included in this section due to the arena of influence in which it finds its application: it is employed for those seeking favor of a jury. While this may be used to promote the causes of justice and honor, it can also be used in rights designed to help the criminal to escape the hands of justice by convincing a jury to decide in his or her favor.

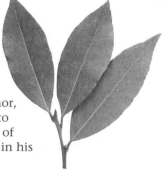

Law Stay Away (v)

hyacinth (MA)
mimosa (mi)
sandalwood (mi)
cinnamon! (T)

> **Background and use:** Another blend designed for the less than honorable element in our society, this magickal preparation is intended for those who are being sought by law enforcement agencies to avoid capture and arrest.

Mystic Veil (v)

sandalwood (MA)
myrrh! (MA)
cinnamon! (T)
clove! (T)

> **Background and use:** The original form of this oil was directed toward more ritual, spiritual purposes. This variation utilizes the facet of the original blend of melding with the world of spirit to more mundane applications. One of the most avid users of this blend is a trucker who drives cross country. He swears that this is what keeps him from getting speeding tickets while trying to keep to stringent deadlines. He says that it acts as a sort of invisibility oil. Highway patrol officers seem to pass right by him without noticing that he is in violation of the speed limit, while they may stop others driving along with him.

No Arrest (v)

patchouli (MA)
cedarwood (MA)
lemon! (mi)
cinnamon! (T)

> **Background and use:** This is another preparation that is popular with those who walk on the shady side of the law. It is designed to help the perpetrator of a criminal offense to avoid being taken into custody by law enforcement officers.

CHAPTER 13

Social Scents

Though many of the most ancient applications of aromatherapy were rooted in therapeutic or magickal concerns, in modern times there is an entire industry related to the social and cosmetic usage of scent. Many of the perfumes and colognes that we see on the market have names that seem to promise love or success, the height of masculine or feminine virtue. They are scents that are named for regal

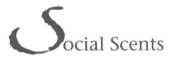

personages, champions, and artistic individuals. They seem to promise wealth, love, and victory.

Is this a hint of the ancient magick at work, or just the work of some clever marketing personnel? Perhaps it is a bit of both. While there is probably little conscious intent on the part of the perfumer to utilize a blend's traditional ingredients to elicit responses embracing the thrill of competitive victory or the realm of the amorous, aromatherapy remains an art of gaining response from the deepest natural instinct. For a product to bring out feelings contrary to its inferred promise—embedded in the name bestowed by the marketing pros—could kill the success and longevity of the commercial offering. Perhaps the most successful blends are the result of both modern marketing techniques as well as the effectiveness of the ancient art of the old magickal cultures.

Today, we treat our homes with scent. We address matters of personal hygiene with fragrance as well as with cleansers and shampoos. We can hardly use any commercial product for the treatment of our bodies or our surroundings without encountering the introduction of aromatherapy into our lives. Floor cleaners, cosmetics, soaps, shampoos, lotions, and even some topical medicines have fragrance added to them. There are products that are aimed strictly at introducing fragrance in our lives, like perfumes, body deodorants, carpet deodorizers, and scented room sprays. Potpourri burners, incense, and scented oil lamps have known some enduring popularity.

There is little evidence that fragrance will disappear anytime soon from the mainstream of our lives or the arena of commercial production. Of the myriad of commercially developed scented products, the formulae included in this section are but a few. Yet they serve as a fine overview of the magnitude and scope of how the world of aromatherapy has permeated the lives of those who may be far from the study of the ancient art or even scoff at the idea that fragrance can have some effect on their daily lives. Many of these same individuals, however, could hardly stand to live with themselves if their dishes were not lemon fresh or if they were to use a fabric softener that did not have the scent of springtime.

Cosmetic Applications

Although there are many uses of fragrance that do not fall under the more ancient practices of magick and healing, the use of scent in cosmetics is one of the most widely enjoyed. And while these applications are not truly a reflection of the antiquity of the art of aromatherapy, they are not without some ties to the ancient practices. Many of the lotions, baths, and cleansers may serve to restore the skin, hair, and general condition of the body to optimum order. Thus, these fragrant applications are not too far removed from healing practices.

Many of the scents used in cosmetic applications are those that evoke pleasant feelings, increase self-appreciation, and, perhaps, elicit the admiration of others. In this respect, they are in tune with the ancient uses of scent in the magickal workings.

The formulas included here are but a sampling of the number of fragrant preparations that may be produced. They form a sound, basic repertoire of cosmetic preparations but can be augmented, adjusted, or improved with the altering of the component scents.

Baby Powder

5–10   drops lavender
2–3   tablespoons cornstarch

Note: When mixing a fine powder like cornstarch with oil, it can be a very messy proposition. The best method for accomplishing this is to mix the components in a plastic sandwich bag, work out the clumps, and you'll end up with a smooth, scented powder.

Baby Oil

5–10   drops lavender
2–3   tablespoons olive oil (or any other carrier oil—refer to appendix for list of carrier oils)

Body Powder—General Formula

30–40   drops essential oil
2–3   tablespoons cornstarch

Body Powder—Individual Formulae

orange! (MA)
lemon! (MA)
patchouli (mi)
cornstarch

rose (MA)
orange! (mi)
cornstarch

bergamot! (MA)
spikenard (mi)
sandalwood (T)
cornstarch

pine (MA)
cedarwood (MA)
juniper (mi)
cornstarch

ylang ylang (MA)
orange! (mi)
clove! (T)
cinnamon! (T)
cornstarch

cypress (MA)
eucalyptus (MA)
sandalwood (MA)
cornstarch

Facial Treatments

Each of the following formulae should be diluted into a carrier oil.

⌐～ *Normal Skin*

lavender (MA)
rose (mi)
jasmine (T)

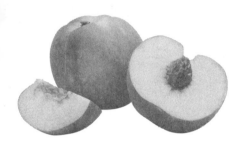

⌐～ *Dry Skin*

sandalwood (MA)
rose (mi)

⌐～ *Oily Skin*

bergamot! (MA)
juniper (mi)
cypress (mi)

Hair Preparations

These base formulae are the pure essential ingredients. To produce a usable hair care product, a total of 24–30 drops of essential oil should be diluted into about 2 tablespoons of carrier oil. The end product can be massaged thoroughly into the hair and scalp. These preparations are similar to the hot oil treatments commercially available for hair care.

⌐～ *Hair Loss*

juniper (MA)
lavender (mi)
rosemary! (mi)

Normal Hair

cedarwood (MA)
bay (MA)
rosemary! (MA)
rose (mi)

Dry Hair

sandalwood (MA)
rose (MA)
lavender (mi)

Oily Hair and Dandruff

ylang ylang (MA)
lime (MA)
rosemary! (mi)

Hand/Skin Care

Dry Hands

benzoin (MA)
rose (MA)
patchouli (MA)

Mouthwashes

Dilute 4–7 drops of oil into a mixture of 4 ounces of water (I prefer distilled water) and 1–1½ teaspoons of honey, depending on the dictates of the individual sweet tooth. A caution: Be certain that the products available from your supplier are certified safe for use in mouthwashes. Not all products may be safe for this application.

Be very careful with this. Check with your supplier before use. While some oils may be safe for internal use, many are not—do not assume that a particular oil is safe without verification from your supplier.

Tart and Minty

lemon! (MA)
spearmint (MA)

Mint Fresh

peppermint! (MA)
spearmint (MA)

A Touch of Spice

spearmint (MA)
orange! (mi)
clove! (mi)

Perfumery

The art of the perfumer, while rooted in antiquity, is full of modern innovations. The old astrological and magickal associations of scent may still be a subtle foundation for the end products that emerge from the perfumer's laboratory. More than likely, however, it is the marketing department of the fragrance vendor that carries on the ancient traditions of the magickal art of aromatherapy.

Perfume names may promise anything from romance to adventure to illicit love. Names evoke visions of the heights of luxury, the depth of passion, or the excitement of living on the edge. The old associations that demand the use of specific scents or combinations of scents for specific purposes may not be apparent in the modern fragrance designer's work. The more modern criteria of olfactory gratification and salability have taken a more prominent role.

Still, the ways of the ancient scent masters are not completely gone from the products of the commercial fragrance factories. One of the things that governs whether a product has enduring salability is the instinctive response by the consumer. While the marketing pros do their best to play up each new scent and ready the buying public to receive it anxiously, it is the gut response of the purchaser that will determine how enduring a product will be. The marketing hype may ensure the first sale—perhaps even the second. In the end, however, the instinctive response of the consumer will determine whether there will be continued use of this product or that. There may be times when the most a product has to offer is the quality of its advertisements.

So, in the end, even those who have forgotten the ancient art of scent are under its influence. The perfume scents offered here are given as popular blends. They are offered with no explanation to use or effect, for they were produced for commercial offering without regard to the ancient artistry of fragrance blending. While many of the blends may parallel some of the magickal preparations for special purpose, their design is likely due more to the delightful effect of the blend and the pleasant instinctive response to the fragrance than because of the perfumer's observation of the principles of the ancient art of aromatherapy. Therefore, the following formulae are offered for educational purposes, for reference examples, and simply for fun and pleasure.

A General Perfume Formula

75–100 drops essential oil or oil blend
¼   fluid ounce of perfumer's alcohol

Low Cost Substitute

75–100 drops essential oil or oil blend
¼   ounce rubbing alcohol

The difference between these two formulae is in the dilution base. Perfumer's alcohol is a mixture of unscented alcohol and glycerin. By far, this is the ideal foundation for a perfume product. However, rubbing alcohol is far less expensive and far more readily available. The major difference is that rubbing alcohol does have a scent of its own—and not a particularly pleasant one, at that! Yet, this is a substitute that can be used successfully if the proper considerations are observed. Although there is an inherent scent to rubbing alcohol, it also evaporates fairly quickly. Once it has evaporated, this will leave the fragrance of the blend as the prominent scent noticeable. However, there is a time factor involved. Where it may be possible to dab on some perfume and run right out to an important engagement, it is wiser to allow some time for the rubbing alcohol substitute to evaporate.

Another difference is that the perfumer's alcohol contains a fixative to bind the mixture. The rubbing alcohol blend may have a tendency to separate and so must be well shaken before use. However, if these considerations are taken into account, the poor man's fragrance is as fine a scent as that produced by the oldest, most respected French perfumery.

Sweet Spice

gardenia (MA)
vetivert (mi)
cinnamon! (T)
pine (T)
clove! (T)

Something Sensuous

ambergris (MA)
jasmine (mi)
musk (mi)
frankincense! (T)

Springtime Freshness

sandalwood (MA)
orange! (MA)
cinnamon! (mi)
rosemary! (T)
lemon verbena! (T)

Lemon Forest

bergamot! (MA)
carnation (mi)
sandalwood (mi)
patchouli (mi)
cedarwood (T)

Sweet Earth Scent

oakmoss! (MA)
bergamot! (mi)
amber (mi)
vetivert (mi)
pine (T)

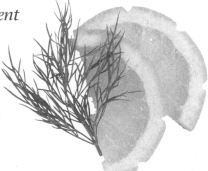

Musky Rose

rose (MA)
musk (mi)
sandalwood (mi)

Floral Bouquet

violet (MA)
heliotrope (mi)
vetivert (mi)
lilac (mi)
juniper (mi)

Nocturnal Mystery

jasmine (MA)
patchouli (MA)
orange! (MA)
vanilla (mi)
amber (mi)

Other Pleasantries

Like the perfume industry, which has diverged from the foundational principles of its ancestral beginnings, fragrance is often used throughout our lives without regard to the associations formulated by the ancient aromatherapy artisans. We look less toward the meanings of certain fragrances and less toward the associations ascribed to each scent by the old scientists and more toward pleasantry. It often matters little whether a fragrance is directed toward love or peace or success, according to the old magickal formulas, but whether it makes our surroundings more appealing, our dwellings more pleasant, and our lives more palatable.

Many of the modern uses of fragrance are not grounded in the ancient practices, but only in individual appeal. These are diverse, and while they have little to do with the practice of aromatherapy, a formulary would seem less than complete without including these common uses of fragrance by modern society.

Mint Fragrance

peppermint! (MA)
spearmint (MA)

Citrus Scent

orangc! (MA)
lemon! (mi)
lime (mi)
bergamot! (T)

Spice Scent

galangal (MA)
vetivert (mi)
cinnamon! (T)
clove! (T)
rosemary! (T)

Floral Scent

jasmine (MA)
rose (mi)
ylang ylang (mi)
benzoin (mi)

Wooded Fragrance

sandalwood (MA)
cypress (mi)
pine (mi)
oakmoss! (mi)
cedarwood (T)

A Kitchen Favorite

orange! (MA)
cinnamon! (T)
clove! (T)

Potpourri

There are many inexpensive potpourri pots available. These are often ceramic and include two compartments—one for the blend of herbs and flowers that comprise the potpourri, and the other for a candle to heat the mixture and disperse the fragrance into the air.

The formulae included above reflect an innovation of the common use of potpourri to scent the home. Although there are many commercially available potpourri mixtures, it is also possible to customize the potpourri to individual taste. This is done by adding a few drops of an oil blend to a base of dried flowers. When set into the potpourri cooker, the oil blend will become the dominant fragrance.

Mist Sprays

There are other uses for this application in the realms of therapeutic and magickal aromatherapy. However, the spray mist may be used simply to introduce a pleasant aroma into the home or office. The preparation is produced by adding 100–125 drops of a favored blend to 4 or 5 ounces of water and placing it in a spray bottle.

Upholstery and Carpet Fresheners

Another household pleasantry that may be concocted from the same delightful oil blends is prepared in powder form. This is done by adding 90–120 drops of an oil blend to about ½ cup of baking soda. Mix the oil well into the powder. Sprinkle the powder on the carpet or furniture fabric. After 15–20 minutes, vacuum the treated area.

Scented Candles

Even those who are not graced with the skill of the candlemaker's trade can produce scented candles for use in the home. One way is to borrow a technique from the books of the old magicians, and anoint the candle with a desired scented oil blend. Another is to interject the scent into the candle. To do this, simply heat a metal ice pick or meat skewer, and melt a hole in the candle. Then place the oil blend in the hole. As the candle burns, the oil will be dispersed into the air, beautifully scenting the home.

Afterword

With the closing pages of this offering comes the hope that a beginning formulary has been faithfully delivered into the hands of those who would pursue the ancient art of aromatherapy. I offer a sound foundation and a basic presentation of the way in which the virtues of fragrance have been realized by the practitioners of this natural science throughout the progressive march of the centuries.

Yet, as complete an overview as is presented here, do not be deceived by its fullness. For in fact what I have done is opened a doorway to the past. The specifics of the formulae are up to the skill and creativity of the individual. This volume is but a guideline to help the creative fragrance artisan along the journey to newer and greater vistas of aromatherapy.

The purpose and the deepest hope accompanying this volume is to instill an awareness and an appreciation of the world of fragrance that surrounds us. In the most basic sense, the aromas that fill the air are gifts of the world of nature. Though we may have accepted the realignment and the repression of many of our natural, inborn systems of response with the acceptance of a commercially dominated world, those instincts lay deep within, waiting for us to recognize and appreciate them once again.

While there is an increased awareness of the defiling of the natural world through the efforts of environmentalists and those who have learned to appreciate the beauty and bounty of nature, there is also the faint echo of the voices of the ancients who knew the secrets that were embodied in the world of nature. In many tongues, through many ages, they call to us to remember.

As we re-educate ourselves in the ways of natural sciences and sorcery, we find that they are interrelated. We also discover that, as we awaken the knowledge of ancient lore, we touch that part of ourselves where inspiration, instinct, and creativity lie waiting to emerge in their fullest glory. As we rediscover the gifts of nature, we also return to that special realm of consciousness where we know ourselves to be a part of the natural world. We touch the seed of life that lies within our own souls and come to the inescapable reality that, within our own beings, we are connected to the greatest of nature's gifts—that of life itself.

The greatest accomplishments are in the hands of a new generation of fragrance explorers: those who travel unafraid to experience new adventures, try new innovations, and offer new insights into an old system of healing and magick. As ancient as the art of fragrance blending may be, historically, it is ever young in its development.

Progress is not measured in the dedication to the detail of the practices of our ancestors. Though we regard the ancient knowledge with respect and all due admiration, the future of the art lies within the hands of the new aromatherapists. From this sound beginning, only the individual artisans of the future will determine how far the art will progress. It is the children of the future that will take the final measure of the ancient art.

PART IV

Appendices

Appendix 1: Planetary Associations

Amber	Jupiter
Ambergris	Venus
Apple	Neptune/Venus
Bay	Sun
Benzoin	Sun/Mercury
Bergamot	Sun
Camphor	Moon
Carnation	Venus/Sun
Cedarwood	Jupiter/Uranus
Cinnamon	Sun
Civet	Venus
Citronella	Sun/Mars
Clove	Jupiter/Sun
Cyclamen	Venus
Cypress	Saturn/Venus
Eucalyptus	Mercury/Saturn
Elderberry	Venus
Frankincense	Sun/Pluto
Galangal	Sun/Mars
Gardenia	Venus/Moon
Heliotrope	Sun
Honeysuckle	Jupiter
Hyacinth	Venus
Jasmine	Jupiter/Moon
Juniper	Sun/Jupiter/Neptune
Lavender	Mercury

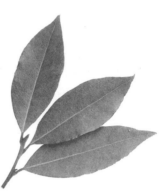

Lemon	Moon
Lemon Verbena	Mercury/Venus
Lilac	Venus/Uranus
Lily of the Valley	Mercury
Lotus	Uranus/Moon
Magnolia	Venus
Mimosa	Saturn/Moon
Muguet	Venus
Musk	Sun/Venus
Myrrh	Sun/Jupiter
Oakmoss	Jupiter
Orange	Sun
Patchouli	Saturn
Peppermint	Mercury
Pine	Mars
Rose	Venus
Rosemary	Sun
Sandalwood	Jupiter/Neptune
Spearmint	Mercury
Spikenard	Saturn/Neptune
Strawberry	Venus
Vanilla	Venus
Vetivert	Jupiter/Uranus
Violet	Venus/Mercury
Wintergreen	Moon
Ylang Ylang	Venus

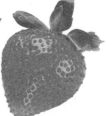

Appendix 2: Astrological Associations

Amber	Libra
Ambergris	Taurus
Apple	Libra
Bay	Aries/Leo
Benzoin	Aries/Gemini
Bergamot	Sagittarius
Camphor	Cancer
Carnation	Aries/Libra
Cedarwood	Aries/Sagittarius
Cinnamon	Leo
Civet	Taurus
Citronella	Aries
Clove	Aries/Sagittarius
Cyclamen	Cancer
Cypress	Libra/Capricorn
Eucalyptus	Gemini/Aquarius
Elderberry	Libra
Frankincense	Leo/Aries
Galangal	Aries/Scorpio
Gardenia	Libra
Heliotrope	Leo/Gemini
Honeysuckle	Cancer
Hyacinth	Taurus/Pisces
Jasmine	Taurus/Cancer
Juniper	Leo/Sagittarius

Lavender	Gemini/Virgo
Lemon	Cancer
Lemon Verbena	Gemini/Virgo
Lilac	Pisces
Lily of the Valley	Gemini/Pisces
Lotus	Aquarius/Cancer
Magnolia	Taurus/Libra
Mimosa	Capricorn/Cancer
Muguet	Libra
Musk	Leo/Sagittarius
Myrrh	Scorpio/Sagittarius
Oakmoss	Taurus
Orange	Leo
Patchouli	Taurus/Capricorn
Peppermint	Gemini
Pine	Aries/Scorpio
Rose	Libra/Cancer
Rosemary	Leo/Aries
Sandalwood	Cancer/Pisces
Spearmint	Gemini
Spikenard	Capricorn/Pisces
Strawberry	Libra
Vanilla	Libra/Pisces
Vetivert	Taurus/Scorpio
Violet	Gemini/Libra
Wintergreen	Cancer
Ylang Ylang	Taurus/Pisces

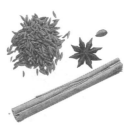

Appendix 3: Elemental Associations

Amber	Earth
Ambergris	Water
Apple	Water
Bay	Fire
Benzoin	Fire
Bergamot	Air/Fire
Camphor	Water
Carnation	Air/Fire
Cedarwood	Air/Earth
Cinnamon	Fire
Civet	Earth/Water
Citronella	Fire
Clove	Fire
Cyclamen	Air/Water
Cypress	Earth/Water
Eucalyptus	Air
Elderberry	Water
Frankincense	Fire
Galangal	Fire
Gardenia	Water/Air
Heliotrope	Fire/Earth
Honeysuckle	Earth/Water
Hyacinth	Water
Jasmine	Water/Earth
Juniper	Fire/Water
Lavender	Air

Lemon	Water
Lemon Verbena	Air
Lilac	Earth
Lily of the Valley	Air/Water
Lotus	Water
Magnolia	Water/Earth
Mimosa	Air/Earth
Muguet	Air/Water
Musk	Earth/Fire
Myrrh	Fire
Oakmoss	Earth
Orange	Fire
Patchouli	Earth
Peppermint	Air
Pine	Earth
Rose	Earth
Rosemary	Fire/Air
Sandalwood	Earth/Water
Spearmint	Air
Spikenard	Water
Strawberry	Air
Vanilla	Water
Vetivert	Earth
Violet	Air
Wintergreen	Earth/Air
Ylang Ylang	Water

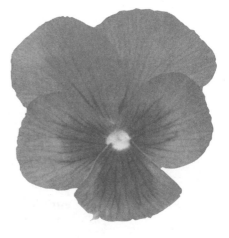

Appendix 4: Gender Associations

Amber	Female
Ambergris	Female
Apple	Female
Bay	Male
Benzoin	Male
Bergamot	Male
Camphor	Female
Carnation	Female
Cedarwood	Male
Cinnamon	Male
Civet	Female
Citronella	Female
Clove	Male
Cyclamen	Female
Cypress	Female
Eucalyptus	Male
Elderberry	Female
Frankincense	Male
Galangal	Male
Gardenia	Female
Heliotrope	Male
Honeysuckle	Male
Hyacinth	Male
Jasmine	Male
Juniper	Male
Lavender	Female

Lemon	Female
Lemon Verbena	Male
Lilac	Female
Lily of the Valley	Female
Lotus	Female
Magnolia	Female
Mimosa	Female
Muguet	Male
Musk	Male
Myrrh	Male
Oakmoss	Male
Orange	Male
Patchouli	Male
Peppermint	Male
Pine	Male
Rose	Female
Rosemary	Male
Sandalwood	Male
Spearmint	Female
Spikenard	Female
Strawberry	Female
Vanilla	Male
Vetivert	Male
Violet	Female
Wintergreen	Male
Ylang Ylang	Female

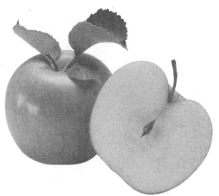

Appendix 5: Magickal Properties

Amber	Healing
Ambergris	Arouse emotion
Apple	Happiness
Bay	Clear sight, energy
Benzoin	Clarity of thought, relief of guilt
Bergamot	Builds self-esteem
Camphor	Calming, shock, awakens past life memories
Carnation	Health, energy
Cedarwood	Cleansing, clears confusion
Cinnamon	Courage, adds energy to other influences
Civet	Female sex scent
Citronella	Cleansing, banishing
Clove	Courage, memory, focus
Cyclamen	Love, peace
Cypress	Comfort, eases losses
Eucalyptus	Openness, health
Elderberry	Joy, arouses emotions
Frankincense	Spirituality, forgiveness of past ills
Galangal	Courage, energy
Gardenia	Love, peace, spirituality
Heliotrope	Health, self-confidence, money drawing
Honeysuckle	Weight loss, self-acceptance
Hyacinth	Love, sleep, legal matters
Jasmine	Love, attraction, overcomes apathy
Juniper	Relieves obsessions
Lavender	Peace, comfort, memory

Lemon	Health, calming, cleansing
Lemon Verbena	Love, instills trust
Lilac	Love, ease
Lily of the Valley	Acceptance, trust
Lotus	Spirituality, love
Magnolia	Arouses sexual pride
Mimosa	Awakens visions
Muguet	Arouses passions
Musk	Animal instinct, sexual desire
Myrrh	Health, spirituality
Oakmoss	Security, stability
Orange	Joy, social interaction
Patchouli	Lifts inhibitions
Peppermint	Clears confusion
Pine	Health, longevity, will to live
Rose	Harmony, eases jealousy
Rosemary	Longevity, memory
Sandalwood	Sexuality, spirituality
Spearmint	Integrity, wisdom
Spikenard	Strength, comfort
Strawberry	Joy, love of life, universal love
Vanilla	Self-confidence, sensuality
Vetivert	Lifts fear and temptation, protection
Violet	Helps alleviate shyness
Wintergreen	Mental and physical well-being
Ylang Ylang	Sex, calming, meditation

Appendix 6: Therapeutic Properties

Amber	General healing
Ambergris	Aphrodisiac properties
Apple	Antidepressant, currently being investigated as an aid in weight loss
Bay	Relaxes muscles, useful for sprains, helps aid breathing, improves digestion, helps to relieve insomnia, promotes perspiration
Benzoin	Stress reducer, reduces congestion, aids in breathing, calming
Bergamot	Helps reduce fatigue as a general tonic, reduces stress, aids in nervous disorders
Camphor	Helps to break up congestion, aids breathing, calming
Carnation	Mood uplifting, boosts energy
Cedarwood	Relaxing, promotes restful sleep, reduces tension
Cinnamon	Pain reliever, aphrodisiac, helps overcome loss of appetite, improves digestion
Civet	Aphrodisiac
Citronella	Insect repellent
Clove	Pain reducer, aphrodisiac, improves digestion, improves mental focus and memory
Cyclamen	Increases metabolism
Cypress	Helps to stabilize irregular menstruation, reduces perspiration, stimulates milk production following childbirth, improves digestion

Eucalyptus	Pain reliever, reduces congestion, aids breathing, reduces fever
Elderberry	Antidepressant
Frankincense	Cough suppressant, calming, aids insomnia
Galangal	Pain reliever, reduces fatigue, improves digestion
Gardenia	Calming, mood uplifting
Heliotrope	General health maintenance, self-confidence
Honeysuckle	Aids in weight loss
Hyacinth	Calming, aids in restful sleep
Jasmine	Aphrodisiac, relieves anxiety and depression, helps reduce cough, aids in treatment of impotence and frigidity
Juniper	Pain reducer, slows inflammation, blood purifier, increases metabolism, reduces gas and stomach disorders, soothing to insect bites
Lavender	Aids in breathing, improves digestion, antidepressant, helpful in skin disorders
Lemon	Fatigue reducer, promotes mental awareness and memory, calming, energizing
Lemon Verbena	Aids in paranoia, helps to instill trust
Lilac	Comforting, relaxing
Lily of the Valley	Aids in memory and mental clarity, promotes self-acceptance
Lotus	Calming, promotes mental clarity and insightful thinking
Magnolia	Aphrodisiac, increases sexual desire
Mimosa	Mood changing, loosens mental rigidity
Muguet	Sexual arousal
Musk	Aphrodisiac

Myrrh	Heals inflammations, helps to regulate menstruation, aids in stomach disorders and loss of appetite
Oakmoss	Instills sense of stability and security
Orange	General health tonic, reduces stress, aids in restful sleep
Patchouli	Stimulating, antidepressant, aids in skin disorders
Peppermint	Pain reliever, energizer, breathing aid, increases appetite, aids in digestion, promotes mental clarity, reduces congestion, reduces hysteria, helpful for headaches (especially due to congestion), reduces fever, beneficial in skin disorders
Pine	Helps relieve breathing difficulties, relieves fatigue, promotes physical strength and endurance, pain reducer
Rose	Calming, pain reducer, aphrodisiac, reduces inflammation, calms nervous stomach
Rosemary	Pain reliever, stimulant, aid to breathing, improves digestion, promotes mental clarity, disinfectant
Sandalwood	Stress reducer, aphrodisiac, healing to the skin, antidepressant, reduces insomnia
Spearmint	Pain reliever, stimulant, improves breathing, soothes itchy skin, refreshing, cooling
Spikenard	Calming, promotes physical strength and endurance, helpful in treating migraines
Strawberry	Mood uplifting, promotes self-acceptance and tolerance
Vanilla	Promotes strength and self-confidence, aids in sexual stamina

Vetivert	Stress reducer, promotes restful sleep, skin healer, pain reliever, promotes physical strength, muscle relaxer
Violet	Promotes self-confidence, helpful in overcoming shyness
Wintergreen	Relief of muscular pain, promotes mental clarity and general health
Ylang Ylang	Muscle relaxer, pain reducer, aphrodisiac, antiseptic, helpful for relief of skin inflammation

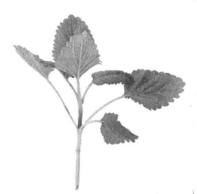

Appendix 7: Therapeutic Cross-References

Analgesic	bergamot, camphor, eucalyptus, lavender, peppermint, rosemary
Antidepressant	bergamot, camphor, elderberry, jasmine, lavender, orange, patchouli, rose, sandalwood, ylang ylang
Antiseptic	bergamot, eucalyptus, juniper, pine
Antispasmodic	bergamot, camphor, cypress, eucalyptus, juniper, lavender, orange, peppermint, rose, rosemary, sandalwood, wintergreen
Antitoxin	juniper, lavender
Aphrodisiac	civet, jasmine, juniper, magnolia, muguet, musk, patchouli, rose, sandalwood, ylang ylang
Astringent	cedarwood, cypress, frankincense, juniper, myrrh, patchouli, peppermint, rose, rosemary, sandalwood
Carminative	benzoin, bergamot, camphor, frankincense, juniper, lavender, myrrh, orange, peppermint, rosemary, sandalwood
Deodorant	benzoin, bergamot, cypress, eucalyptus, lavender, orange, patchouli
Digestive	bergamot, frankincense, orange, rosemary
Diuretic	benzoin, camphor, cedarwood, cypress, eucalyptus, frankincense, juniper, lavender, rosemary, sandalwood
Expectorant	benzoin, bergamot, cedarwood, eucalyptus, myrrh, peppermint, sandalwood
Hypertensor	camphor, rosemary

Hypotensor	lavender, orange, ylang ylang
Laxative	camphor, rose
Nervine	juniper, lavender, lemon verbena, orange, peppermint, rosemary
Sedative	benzoin, bergamot, camphor, cedarwood, cypress, frankincense, jasmine, juniper, lavender, lemon, myrrh, orange, patchouli, rose, sandalwood, ylang ylang
Stimulant	camphor, carnation, eucalyptus, galangal, orange, peppermint, rosemary
Stomachic	juniper, myrrh, orange, peppermint, rose, rosemary
Tonic	bergamot, camphor, carnation, cypress, frankincense, jasmine, juniper, lavender, myrrh, orange, patchouli, rose, sandalwood
Vasoconstrictor	cypress, peppermint
Vulnerary	benzoin, bergamot, camphor, eucalyptus, frankincense, juniper, lavender, myrrh, rosemary

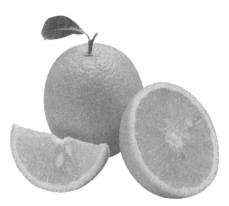

Appendix 8: Magickal Properties

Business	hyacinth, jasmine, patchouli
Cleansing	cedarwood, clove, lemon, lime, pine
Confidence	benzoin, bergamot, honeysuckle, patchouli, vanilla
Courage	cinnamon, galangal
Court Cases	hyacinth, jasmine, oakmoss, patchouli
Energy	bay, carnation, cinnamon, elderberry, galangal, orange
Happiness	apple, honeysuckle, lime
Healing	amber, lemon, myrrh, pine, rosemary, wintergreen
Insight	bay, Lily of the Valley, peppermint, violet, ylang ylang
Joy	eucalyptus, elderberry, orange, strawberry
Love	gardenia, hyacinth, jasmine, lemon verbena, lilac, lotus, rose, ylang ylang
Money Drawing	heliotrope, patchouli, vanilla
Past Lives	camphor, magnolia, mimosa, ylang ylang
Peace	cypress, gardenia, juniper, lavender, lemon, lilac, Lily of the Valley, rose, ylang ylang
Prosperity	heliotrope, jasmine, patchouli, vanilla
Protection	oakmoss, patchouli, vetivert
Sex	ambergris, civet, magnolia, muguet, musk, patchouli, rose, sandalwood, vanilla, ylang ylang
Sleep	cypress, hyacinth, lavender, rose

Spirituality	frankincense, gardenia, lotus, myrrh, sandalwood
Strength	cinnamon, galangal, spikenard, wintergreen
Visions	elderberry, jasmine, mimosa, violet, ylang ylang

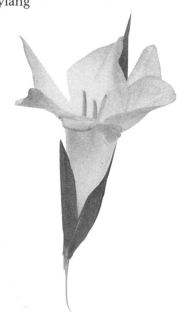

Appendix 9: Magickal Cross-References

Aunt Ana Wishbone	*see*	Fantasy
Banishing	*see*	Needed Changes
Bewitching	*see*	Controlling Oil
Black Candle Tobacco	*see*	Just Judge
Bruno's Curse	*see*	Protection
Bull Oil	*see*	Minoan Oil
Candle	*see*	Holy Oil
Cleo May	*see*	Come to Me
Conjure Oil	*see*	Obeah
Commanding	*see*	Controlling Oil
Desire Me	*see*	Come to Me
Exodus	*see*	Get Away
God	*see*	Divine Man
Goddess	*see*	Divine Woman
Goddess of Love	*see*	Enchantment
Goona Goona	*see*	Sesame Customer Attraction
Haitian Gambler	*see*	Gambler's Oil
Holy Spirit	*see*	Blessing Oil
Honey	*see*	Stay at Home
Hot Foot	*see*	Get Away
Hypnotic Oil	*see*	Meditation
Invisible	*see*	Mystic Veil
Jamaica Bush	*see*	Gambler's Oil
Japanese	*see*	Holy Oil
Lucky Planet	*see*	Prosperity
Manpower	*see*	All Night Long

Appendix 10: Irritant Oils

While there are many oils that may be irritating to more highly sensitive individuals, some are almost universally and to a greater degree likely to cause discomfort. These are marked with a (!) in the text to accentuate that the greatest amount of caution should be exercised.

Anise	Lemon
Bergamot	Lemongrass
Camphor	Lemon Verbena
Cassia	Melissa
Cayenne	Myrrh
Chili Pepper	Oakmoss
Cinnamon	Orange
Citronella	Peppermint
Clove	Rosemary
Frankincense	Wintergreen

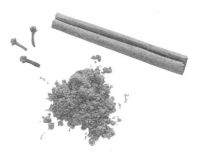

Appendix 11: Carrier Oils

Almond	Hazelnut	Safflower
Apricot	Jojoba	Sesame
Calendula	Olive	Soybean
Corn	Palm	Sunflower
Grape seed	Peanut	Walnut

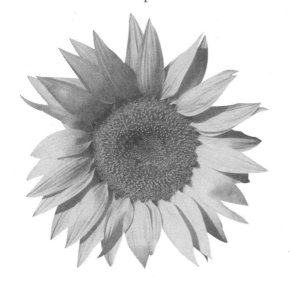

Appendix 12: Oil Sources

There have been many different suppliers that I have had the opportunity to try. While many are excellent sources, there is one that has consistently surpassed expectations in both quality and consistency, which is:

Standard Aromatics
621 West 130th Street
New York, NY 10027
(212) 926-2000

For convenience and location, several other oil sources have been listed. While I deal almost exclusively with Standard Aromatics, some of the other listed enterprises may be more convenient or preferable to other individuals.

M & R Enterprises
15500 Erwin St. #2463
Van Nuys, CA 91411
(800) 324-2284

Liberty National Products
8120 SE Stark Street
Portland, OR 97215
(800) 289-8427

Aroma Vera
3384 S. Robertson Place
Culver City, CA 90034
(800) 669-9514

Leydet Aromatics
P.O. Box 2354
Fair Oaks, CA 95628
(916) 965-7546

Essential Products of America
5018 N. Hubert Ave.
Tampa, FL 33614
(800) 822-9698

Original Swiss Aromatics
P.O. Box 606
San Rafael, CA 94915

As far as retail and/or mail order oil products are concerned, these are just a few of the shops I have personally found impressive:

L'Eclipse Essentials
P.O. Box 13608
Arlington, TX 76094-0608

San Judas (habla espãnol!)
111 W. 6th Street
Irving, TX 75061
(972) 254-1174

Scorpio Herbs
2922 Oaklawn
Dallas, TX 75219
(214) 528-2148

White Light Pentacles/Sacred Spirit Products
P.O. Box 8163
Salem, MA 01971-8163

Glossary

Allopathic medicine	A system of healing utilizing remedies that combats ailments through reversal of symptomatic characteristics of the disease treated.
Analgesic	Pain relieving.
Anointing oil	Singular oil or blend utilized in sacred ritual to dress candles or other ritual trappings, or the body of the practitioner.
Anti-nervine	A remedy used to combat nervous disorders.
Antidepressant	Spirit lifting, counteracting sensations of melancholy.
Antiseptic	Cleansing, combating the growth or spread of bacteria.
Antispasmodic	Acting to relieve muscle spasm.
Antitoxin	Counteracts poisoning.
Aphrodisiac	Heightens sexual desires.
Aromatic sense	Phrase denoting the responsible working of the aromatherapy principles with awareness, reason, and compassion.
Astringent	Causes tightening of skin or tissues.
Candle magick	Utilizing candles as representing units of influence to accomplish a given exercise of will through sorcery.
Carminative	Eases stomach pains and gas.
Carrier oils	These are oils of low scent or no scent used to dilute more pungently aromatic oils or blends.
Chakras	Spiritual centers as practiced in Tantra.

Deodorant	Counteracts body odor.
Digestive	Aids in the digestive system.
Direct inhalation	Breathing fragrant oils directly, without the employment of a medium.
Distillation	The process of boiling or steaming raw materials in order to extract essential oils through cooling and condensation.
Diuretic	Encourages the secretion of urine; a liquid purging of the system.
Elemental association	Each essential aroma may be recognized as being under the influence of the four cardinal energies of the universe: Earth, Air, Fire, and Water.
Enfleurage	An extraction method in which the raw materials are sealed up with a base oil. The process is repeated again and again until the base oil is infused with the aroma of the host.
Essential oil	The aromatic oil that exists naturally and can be extracted from various plants.
Evaporation	An extraction method in which solvents are employed to dissolve a host plant. The solvent is then boiled off. The remaining material includes the essence of the plant.
Expectorant	Raises, helps to expel phlegm.
Expression	This method of oil extraction employs the exertion of pressure on the raw material to squeeze out the essential oil.
Floor wash	A mixture used to cleanse the household. With the inclusion of appropriate aroma blends, this can be used to enhance any predetermined magickal intention.
Formulary	A collection of essential oil blends used as a guidebook for the aromatherapist. A recipe book for the oil mixologist.

Fragrance magick	Magickal aromatherapy using fragrance to accomplish acts of will.
Herbology	The study and use of plant life for medicinal and/or magickal purposes.
Hex oil	An aromatic blend used in magick for the purpose of bringing ill fortune on the subject of the rite.
Homeopathy	A system of treatment utilizing minute doses of substances that would, in a healthy subject, create the symptoms of the ailment being treated.
Humidifier	A device originally designed to deliver moisture to the air, sometimes used by the aromatherapist to fill the air with scent.
Hypertensor	Increases blood pressure.
Hypotensor	Decreases blood pressure.
Incense	A mixture of herbs, plants, and/or essential oils in a flower or wood base that, when burned, is aromatic. Incense has been used for centuries in religious and magickal rites.
Indirect inhalation	To breathe in the scent of a blended oil by delivering the scent first to a carrier medium, like the air.
Infusion	Steeping or soaking a substance in a medium such as water or a carrier oil to extract its virtues.
Irritant oils	Those oils that are commonly offensive or invasive to the skin or the nostrils. While these are sometimes employed in aromatherapy, they are often used only in the smallest quantities and only with the greatest of caution.
Laxative	Promotes bowel activity.

Light ring	A circular device often constructed of brass with a cotton linen insert or of a porous material such as clay. It is placed over a light bulb, filled with fragrant oil, and utilized to deliver scent to the air with the aid of the bulb's heat.
Maceration	A method of extraction in which a plant is crushed and added to a carrier oil. This is repeated until a desired fragrance level is reached. The oil is then drained and applied in aromatherapy.
Magick	The use of natural energies in order to effect a physical change. Spelled with a "k" to differentiate it from stage magic.
Magickal application	To use in connection with a non-physical intention to bring about a change in a life situation.
Major element	The influence (Earth, Air, Fire, or Water) that exerts the greatest influence on, or is most apparent in, an essential oil.
Massage therapy	Utilizing the manipulation of muscles and tissues for healing purposes. This is done through kneading, rubbing, tapping, or stroking with the hands in a prescribed manner.
Minor element	The influence (Earth, Air, Fire, or Water) that is acting upon or characteristic of an essential oil in a secondary capacity.
Natural magick	Utilizing the energies apparent within ourselves and the world around us to effect a physical change in a condition or life situation.
Nervine	Used for general nervous disorders.

New Age	A catch-all term for the revival, revitalization, and augmentation of the old arts and sciences tied with natural healing, magick, and self-awareness.
Oil association	The influence or influences apparent within an essential oil. These may be along the lines of gender, elemental, or planetary.
Oil diffuser	A machine that is specially designed as a system of delivering fragrances from an oil or oil blend into the air.
Pheromones	One of several hormones secreted during arousal as a prelude to sexual activities. These have specific scents that attract the opposite sex, which can be re-created through aromatherapy.
Planetary association	Influence exerted on or apparent in an essential oil in accordance with astrological practice and legendry.
Potpourri	A combination of different aromatic substances generally heated to infuse the air with a pleasing aromatic blend.
Santería	Strictly translated, it means "the worship of the saints." It is a system of religious belief and magickal practice employed largely in Africa, Mexico, South America, and the Caribbean.
Scented waters	Water into which an aromatic dilution of essential fragrance has been introduced.
Sedative	Has a calming effect; sometimes used to allay stress in order to permit restful sleep.
Smoking	An ancient method of healing where aromatic herbs are burned in order to deliver the virtues of their fragrance to an ailing subject.

Solvent	A liquid substance capable of dissolving or dispersing other substances. In the practice of aromatherapy, benzene and alcohol are commonly used.
Spray mist	A scented water (usually a combination of water, alcohol, and essential oil) used to deliver fragrance to the air for therapeutic or magickal purpose.
Sprinkling powders	An aromatic substance blending into a fine base used for the transference of the magickal virtues of a given scent to a given location by dusting the area with the substance.
Stimulant	Raises energy levels.
Stomachic	A stomach tonic used for the relief of stomach disorders.
Synthetic scent	A re-creation of a natural fragrance utilizing sources other than that from which the scent would derive in nature.
Therapeutic application	Use in healing or treatment of ailments or disorders.
Three-circle system	A system of testing the responsibility level of a magickal operation before entering into it.
Tonic	Invigorating, energizing.
Topical dressings	Treatments that are applied externally to an affected area.
Trace element	A minute amount of an ingredient used in the creation of an oil blend (usually only a drop or two).
Vaporizer	A device used for converting liquid to gaseous form for inhalation.
Vasoconstrictor	Causes constriction of capillaries, used to slow blood flow.

Voodoo   A system of religio-magickal practice that
          originated in Africa. It is currently also
          practiced widely in Haiti. In the United
          States, New Orleans is readily recognized
          as a Voodoo center.

Vulnerary Used to heal cuts, sores, and open wounds.

Yang   The masculine, active principle in nature
          that is derived from Oriental philosophy
          and cosmology.

Yin   The female, passive principle of Oriental
          teachings that acts as a complement and
          completion of Yang.

Bibliography

Culpeper, Nicholas. *Culpeper's Complete Herbal & English Physician*. Deansgate, Manchester, England: J. Gleave and Son, 1826. Reproduced by Harvey Sales, 1981.

Cunningham, Scott. *Magical Aromatherapy*. St. Paul, Minn.: Llewellyn Publications, Inc., 1990.

Forey, Pamela and Ruth Lindsay. *Medicinal Plants*. Avenel, N.J.: Atlantis Publications Ltd./ Crescent Books/ Outlet Book Company, Inc., 1991.

Greer, Mary K. *The Essence of Magic*. Van Nuys, Calif.: Newcastle Publishing Company, Inc., 1993.

Heinerman, John. *Science of Herbal Medicine*. Orem, Utah: Bi-World Publishers, 1984.

Lampe, H. U. *Famous Voodoo Rituals and Spells*. Minneapolis, Minn.: Marlar Publishing Company, 1974.

Leek, Sybil. *Sybil Leek's Book of Herbs*. New York, N.Y.: Cornerstone Library, 1980.

Lust, John. *The Herb Book*. New York, NY: Bantam, published by arrangement with Benedict Lust Publications, 1974.

Pelton, Robert W. *Voodoo Charms and Talismans*. New York, N.Y.: Drake Publishers, Inc., 1973.

Riggs, Maribeth. *The Scented Woman*. New York, N.Y.: Viking Studio Books, published by the Penguin Group, 1992.

Riva, Anna. *Golden Secrets of Mystic Oils*. Toluca Lake, Calif.: International Imports, 1978.

Rose, Jeanne. *The Aromatherapy Book*. Berkeley, Calif.: North Atlantic Books, 1992.

Schiller, Carol and David. *500 Formulas For Aromatherapy*. New York, N.Y.: Sterling Publishing Company, Inc., 1994.

Slater, Herman. *Magickal Formulary, Volume One*. New York, N.Y.: Magickal Childe Publishing, Inc., 1981.

Tisserand, Robert B. *The Art of Aromatherapy*. New York, N.Y.: Inner Traditions International Ltd., 1977.

Index of Magickal Blends

Index of Therapeutic Blends

General Index

☾ LOOK FOR THE CRESCENT MOON

Llewellyn publishes hundreds of books on your favorite subjects! To get these exciting books, including the ones on the following pages, check your local bookstore or order them directly from Llewellyn.

ORDER BY PHONE

- Call toll-free within the U.S. and Canada, 1-800-THE MOON
- In Minnesota, call (612) 291-1970
- We accept VISA, MasterCard, and American Express

ORDER BY MAIL

- Send the full price of your order (MN residents add 7% sales tax) in U.S. funds, plus postage & handling to:

  Llewellyn Worldwide
  P.O. Box 64383, Dept. K348-4
  St. Paul, MN 55164–0383, U.S.A.

POSTAGE & HANDLING

(For the U.S., Canada, and Mexico)

- $4.00 for orders $15.00 and under
- $5.00 for orders over $15.00
- No charge for orders over $100.00

We ship UPS in the continental United States. We ship standard mail to P.O. boxes. Orders shipped to Alaska, Hawaii, The Virgin Islands, and Puerto Rico are sent first-class mail. Orders shipped to Canada and Mexico are sent surface mail.

International orders: Airmail—add freight equal to price of each book to the total price of order, plus $5.00 for each non-book item (audio tapes, etc.).

Surface mail—Add $1.00 per item.

Allow 4–6 weeks for delivery on all orders.
Postage and handling rates subject to change.

DISCOUNTS

We offer a 20% discount to group leaders or agents. You must order a minimum of 5 copies of the same book to get our special quantity price.

FREE CATALOG

Get a free copy of our color catalog, *New Worlds of Mind and Spirit.* Subscribe for just $10.00 in the United States and Canada ($30.00 overseas, airmail). Many bookstores carry *New Worlds*—ask for it!

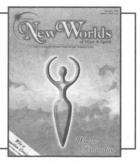

Visit our website at www.llewellyn.com for more information.

Pagan Ways
Finding Your Spirituality in Nature

Gwydion O'Hara

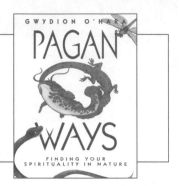

Do you feel the spirituality in nature? Are you full of questions about mainstream religion? Do you long to engage in rituals that have meaning for you? Perhaps you are a Pagan at heart.

Pagan Ways is your first step toward finding your personal spiritual truth. It is designed to offer enough understanding and insight to allow a fully thought-out and firm decision as to whether Paganism is, indeed, the path for you.

Explore the history of Paganism and the founders of the modern Craft movement. Learn how the Pagan God is found in the cycles of the seasons, how to get in touch with nature spirits, what celebrations are included in the Pagan calendar, the tools used for magick and worship, how to erect an altar, how to conduct a ritual, how the eight Pagan virtues fit into your life, and what the stages are to becoming a Priest or Priestess.

1-56718-341-7
5³⁄₁₆ x 8, 216 pp. $7.95

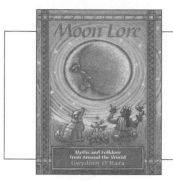

Moon Lore
Myths & Folklore from
Around the World

Gwydion O'Hara

Most of us love stories. But the rich messages spun in folklore—especially in oral traditions—are not found in the media from which we get most of our knowledge today. Fairytales rehashed in mega-productions like "Beauty and the Beast" don't often serve the true function of a fairy or folktale. Where are the stories that entertain, enlighten and bring us all closer together?

Moon Lore is a collection of original tales all about the people of many lands and times. The one common thread connecting the stories is the Moon: the heavenly body that has guided humankind since the beginning of time. Today Moon mythology continues to bind the people of the world together, reflecting our diverse lives in all her faces. *Moon Lore*'s magical characters and settings spring to life in tales of jealousy, fear, triumph, celebration, love and challenge. Find out what the Hindi Wisemen see in the Moon (it's not a man's face). Jack and Jill are in *Moon Lore*, but in this Germanic variation, magic brew is what they fetch, and they never tumble down the hill! Chapters are divided into 13 segments, each lunar month presenting a new myth from Celtic, Chinese, Native American and other traditions and cultures.

1-56718-342-5
5¼ x 8, 256 pp., index, softcover $9.95

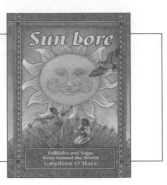

Sun Lore

*Folktales and Sagas from
Around the World*

Gwydion O'Hara

Tales of simplicity and glory ... death and life ... compassion and devastation—there is little that has not been within the reaches of the Sun. From the beginning of time, when getting through each new day was an end in itself, the sun watched overhead.

Sun Lore is a bridge between the primitive man who lived and worshipped according to those things that were beyond understanding, and the modern man of reason who attempts to analyze the world in which we live. The fifty illustrated tales are a celebration of the sun worshippers of ancient times, offered up for the insight and enjoyment of their descendants who dwell in an age of science.

Read stories from around the world about the creation of life, about how each sun god and goddess came to be, and folktales about the Sun as hero and fool. In experiencing the old legends of Father Sun, we can realign ourselves with the forgotten times that hold the roots of our modern existence, and that shape our families, faith and cultures

1-56718-343-3
5¼ x 8, 224 pp., softcover   **$9.95**

To order, call 1-800-THE MOON
Prices subject to change without notice

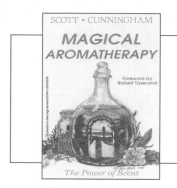

Magical Aromatherapy
The Power of Scent

Scott Cunningham

Scent magic has a rich, colorful history. Today, in the shadow of the next century, there is much we can learn from the simple plants that grace our planet. Most have been used for countless centuries. The energies still vibrate within their aromas.

Scott Cunningham has now combined the current knowledge of the physiological and psychological effects of natural fragrances with the ancient art of magical perfumery. In writing this book, he drew on extensive experimentation and observation, research into 4,000 years of written records, and the wisdom of respected aromatherapy practitioners. *Magical Aromatherapy* contains a wealth of practical tables of aromas of the seasons, days of the week, the planets, and zodiac; use of essential oils with crystals; synthetic and genuine oils and hazardous essential oils. It also contains a handy appendix of aromatherapy organizations and distributors of essential oils and dried plant products.

0-87542-129-6
mass market, 224 pp., illus. $3.95

To order, call 1-800-THE MOON
Prices subject to change without notice

The Complete Book of Incense, Oils & Brews

Scott Cunningham

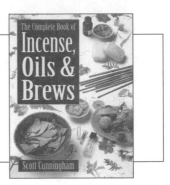

For centuries the composition of incenses, the blending of oils, and the mixing of herbs have been used by people to create positive changes in their lives. With this book, the curtains of secrecy have been drawn back, providing you with practical, easy-to-understand information that will allow you to practice these methods of magical cookery.

Scott Cunningham, world-famous expert on magical herbalism, first published *The Magic of Incense, Oils & Brews* in 1986. *The Complete Book of Incense, Oils & Brews* is a revised and expanded version of that book. Scott took readers' suggestions from the first edition and added more than 100 new formulas. Every page has been clarified and rewritten, and new chapters have been added.

There is no special, costly equipment to buy, and ingredients are usually easy to find. The book includes detailed information on a wide variety of herbs, sources for purchasing ingredients, substitutions for hard-to-find herbs, a glossary, and a chapter on creating your own magical recipes.

0-87542-128-8
6 x 9, 288 pp., illus., softcover $12.95

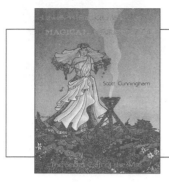

Magical Herbalism
The Secret Craft of the Wise

Scott Cunningham

Certain plants are prized for the special range of energies—the vibrations, or powers—they possess. *Magical Herbalism* unites the powers of plants and man to produce, and direct, change in accord with human will and desire.

This is the Magic of amulets and charms, sachets and herbal pillows, incenses and scented oils, simples and infusions and anointments. It's Magic as old as our knowledge of plants, an art that anyone can learn and practice, and once again enjoy as we look to the Earth to rediscover our roots and make inner connections with the world of Nature. This is Magic that is beautiful and natural—a Craft of Hand and Mind merged with the Power and Glory of Nature: a special kind that does not use the medicinal powers of herbs, but rather the subtle vibrations and scents that touch the psychic centers and stir the astral field in which we live to work at the causal level behind the material world.

This is Magic for everyone—for the herbs are easily and readily obtained, the tools are familiar or easily made, and the technology that of home and garden. This book includes step-by-step guidance to the preparation of herbs and to their compounding in incense and oils, sachets and amulets, simples and infusions, with simple rituals and spells for every purpose.

0-87542-120-2
5¼ x 8, 260 pp., illus., softcover $9.95

Mother Nature's Herbal

Judy Griffin, Ph.D.

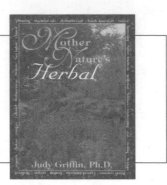

A Zuni American Indian swallows the juice of goldenrod flowers to ease his sore throat … an East Indian housewife uses the hot spices of curry to destroy parasites … an early American settler rubs fresh strawberry juice on her teeth to remove tartar. People throughout the centuries have enjoyed a special relationship with Nature and her many gifts. Now, with *Mother Nature's Herbal*, you can discover how to use a planet full of medicinal and culinary herbs through more than 200 recipes and tonics. Explore the cuisine, beauty secrets and folk remedies of China, the Mediterranean, South America, India, Africa and North America. The book will also teach you the specific uses of flower essences, chakra balancing, aromatherapy, essential oils, companion planting, organic gardening and theme garden designs.

1-56718-340-9
7 x 10, 448 pp., 16-page color insert, softcover $19.95

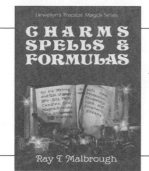

Charms, Spells & Formulas

For the Making and Use of Gris-Gris Bags,
Herb Candles, Doll Magic,
Incenses, Oils, and Powders

Ray Marlbrough

Hoodoo magick is a blend of European techniques and the magick brought to the New World by slaves from Africa. Now you can learn the methods that have been used successfully by Hoodoo practitioners for nearly 200 years.

By using the simple materials available in nature, you can bring about the necessary changes to greatly benefit your life and that of your friends. You are given detailed instructions for making and using the "gris-gris" (charm) bags only casually or mysteriously mentioned by other writers. Malbrough not only shows how to make gris-gris bags for health, money, luck, love and protection from evil and harm, but he also explains how these charms work. He also takes you into the world of doll magick to gain love, success, or prosperity. Complete instructions are given for making the dolls and setting up the ritual.

0-87542-501-1
5¼ x 8, 192 pp., illus., softcover $6.95

Aromatherapy

Balance the Body and Soul
with Essential Oils

Ann Berwick

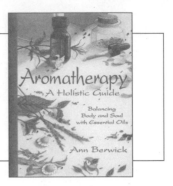

For thousands of years, aromatherapy—the therapeutic use of the essential oils of aromatic plants—has been used for the benefit of mankind. These oils are highly concentrated forms of herbal energy that represent the soul, or life force, of the plant. When the aromatic vapor is inhaled, it can influence areas of the brain inaccessible to conscious control such as emotions and hormonal responses. Application of the oils in massage can enhance the benefits of body work on the muscular, lymphatic and nervous systems. By cutaneous application of the oils, we can influence more deeply the main body systems.

This is the first complete guide to holistic aromatherapy—what it is, how and why it works. Written from the perspective of a practicing aromatherapist, *Aromatherapy* provides insights into the magic of creating body balance through the use of individually blended oils, and it offers professional secrets of working with these potent substances on the physical, mental, emotional and spiritual levels.

0-87542-033-8
6 x 9, 240 pp., illus., softcover $12.95

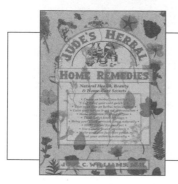

Jude's Herbal Home Remedies
Natural Health, Beauty & Home-Care Secrets

Jude C. Williams, M.H.

There's a pharmacy—in your spice cabinet! In the course of daily life we all encounter problems that can be easily remedied through the use of common herbs—headaches, dandruff, insomnia, colds, muscle aches, burns—and a host of other afflictions known to humankind. *Jude's Herbal Home Remedies* is a simple guide to self care that will benefit beginning or experienced herbalists with its wealth of practical advice. Most of the herbs listed are easy to obtain.

Discover how cayenne pepper promotes hair growth, why cranberry juice is a good treatment for asthma attacks, how to make a potent juice to flush out fat, how to make your own deodorants and perfumes, what herbs will get fleas off your pet, how to keep cut flowers fresh longer ... the remedies and hints go on and on!

This book gives you instructions for teas, salves, tinctures, tonics, poultices, along with addresses for obtaining the herbs. Dangerous and controversial herbs are also discussed.

Grab this book and a cup of herbal tea, and discover from a Master Herbalist more than 800 ways to a simpler, more natural way of life.

0-87542-869-X
6 x 9, 240 pp., illus., softcover $12.95